Before me is the Door

David Fischer MD PhD

DEDICATION

For Håkon...
.

I was nothing, no one, I was everything to her, I was hers.
~Sharon Olds, The Wellspring...

CHAPTER ONE

Tuesday, July 3, 1984

Before me is the door to the single dorm room. I stand quietly before it. It's late. Bubbles is probably sleeping, but still I have to knock so I don't embarrass her. I feel guilty - She's probably had a hard day and now I have to wake her.

I knock on the door. There's no answer. I rush into the room and a burst of light enters with me. Quickly I close the door, but keep it a crack open. I can barely see the bed and can't distinguish whether anyone is in there. Then I see her.

"Bubbles," I say.

"Hi Davy!" she says in excited tones.

"I'm sorry I woke you, Bubbles. I had to stay at the lab till late."

"What were you doing?"

I sat on the edge of the bed.

"I wanted to attempt another method of solving a crystal structure."

"Oh. What time is it?"

"12:30. I'm sorry, Bubbles."

"That's okay."

"How was your first day with that vet school student at the hospital?"

"It was okay - I got lost." She pulled herself up on the bed as her tone became more excited. "We were walking with a horse when she told me to wait for her while she did something else for a minute. So she left - And, Davy, she didn't come back!"

She burst into laughter.

"Where did she go?"

"I don't know. She just left me with that horse. Finally I followed around another guy on his rounds. Then I saw her... It was funny. First days are always like that."

"Yeah, first days are tough."

I hesitated.

"Bubbles, you know what?... This whole weekend I'd been worrying that the X-ray diffractometer wasn't going to work because of something I did on Saturday. I turned a switch, and, Bubbles, I wasn't sure it was the right one. I thought I'd messed up the whole system. All I could hear in my ears - I mean from my conscience - was Professor Hope telling me, 'Dave, fuck you. Fuck you, Dave. Get out of here. Go home.' I swear, Bubbles, this whole weekend I was worried about what was going to happen when that X-ray diffractometer was turned on. And you know what?... Professor Poole turned it on today, and there wasn't a thing wrong with it."

"David, you worry too much."

"It was a stupid thing to do. When am I going to learn not to touch things if I'm not sure how to really use them? Now, every time I do do something like that - or even think about it – I hear that Norwegian accent in the back of my mind saying, 'Fuck you, Mike. Fuck you. Go home.'"

"It's really drilled into you, isn't it?"

"Bubbles, no matter what I do or where I go or how much time passes, I'll always hear those words - I'll hear them for the rest of my life."

"David, you're too much."

Lying beside her, I put my head on her shoulder.

"Bubbles, you know who I saw today?"

"Who?"

She turned on her side and looked at me.

"I saw that my old TA [Teaching Assistant] for Organic Chemistry. He was bringing his bike up the stairway when he stopped and asked me what the Hell I was doing here? I told him I came back to continue my research in X-ray diffraction."

I laughed.

"Bubbles, he says to me, 'You should be in some exotic land chasing wild women.' I told him that I had been when I was in Florida, but came back when Professor Hope told me his achievement in determining the molecular structure of a protein. He said I was too dedicated."

"You are, Dave."

I looked up to the ceiling.

"A couple of days ago I really pissed Brendan off," I confided. "I was on the X-ray diffractometer and something happened that I wasn't sure I could fix. So I called him up and got him in there at midnight. The next day I found out how mad he was. He comes in and tells me that if I want to use the X-ray diffractometer anymore when no one's around, it's my ass if anything goes wrong. 'I'm not here to serve you, David. I tell you things and you don't listen.' Damn it, Brendan, I'm sorry. I know how to fix that camera, I just didn't trust my hands. I never did it before, Bubbles. I wasn't sure I could do it without damaging it."

"I'm like that, too, Dave. I just don't know how to do something until I've done it myself."

"I swear, Bubbles, if I had one wish - One wish..."

"You wouldn't have called," she inserted.

"No, no. I don't regret the things that have happened," I responded. "If I had one wish I'd wish that one day I could see Brendan and smile and say 'Hi, Brendan', and he would smile and say, 'Hi Dave.' But it will never happen. He's the teacher and I'm the student. I walk in there and Brendan will look up and say, 'Yes, David, what is it now?'"

"He sounds like an unhappy person. It's hard to learn from people who don't have enthusiasm."

"No, Bubbles. Brendan is a good guy. It's me. I've been working in X-ray diffraction for a whole year, but I haven't studied it like I should because I've been so pre-occupied with my studies. All the time Brendan was there to help me. Now, he's had it. Fed up.. Sick of it. Sick of me. And the worse thing is, I really like him and I've appreciated his help. You should have seen, Bubbles - The day he got mad at me, I went out and bought him a box of Pepperidge Farm cookies. I was going to give it to him as a peace offering. But I was too late; he'd already left for a trip to New Jersey. I still have the cookies in my lab. It reminds me of how bad I feel about not learning as much as I should have from him."

"David, you're too hard on yourself. You shouldn't be. You work hard and you never mean to make mistakes. The things you feel bad about are always accidents. You never mean to hurt anyone." Her voice trailed off. "I remember once - Oh, I was so bad. I hate losing friends, and this time I was just evil."

"What did you do, Bubbles?"

"No, I can't tell you, David."

"Com'on, Bubbles. Get it off your chest. You wouldn't have brought it up if you didn't want to tell someone."

"No, it's the worst thing I've ever done. I can't talk about it."

"Bubbles, it can't even be half as bad as some of the things I've done. Could it be that bad?"

"David, you didn't mean to hurt anyone. I really wanted to hurt this other girl. It was terrible."

"Tell me, Bubbles."

"No, Dave. I'd be too embarrassed."

She got out of the bed and went out into the hallway. I laid on the bed waiting for her.

Returning to the room, sat on the bed next to me, then set the alarm clock on the dresser.

I got off the bed and prepared a place to sleep on the floor.

"I'm tired, Bubbles. I'm going to bed."

"You sure you don't want to sleep on the bed, David?"

"Yes, Bubbles."

"I like sleeping on the floor, Davy..."

"No, Bubbles," I insisted. "Goodnight..."

CHAPTER TWO

Thursday, July 4, 1984

I've just spent the entire day in the lab working on the X-ray diffractometer. As of yet I've been unsuccessful - failure, crystal after crystal. Either I'm not quick enough in getting the crystal on and they begin to decompose. Or else the crystal is twinned or cracked, and unsatisfactory.

It's 7:30 PM. Today is the Fourth of July. Bubbles and I are supposed to watch the fireworks. I telephoned her from the lab.

"Hello."

"Hi Bubbles."

"Hi David."

"Bubbles, let's go to the fireworks."

"Are you busy, David?"

"Yes, but the crystals aren't very good, and I want to go."

"You sure."

"Yes. Come on over. I'm finished."

"Is everything alright, Davy?"

I hesitated.

"We failed. A day wasted." I let out a sigh. "I'll meet you outside the Chem Building."

"Bye, Davy."

I went back to the X-ray room. I looked at the crystals through the polarizing microscope.

"How can something so beautiful be so much trouble?" I thought.

I went outside and unlocked my bike. I began riding to Bubbles', then saw her riding up. She was wearing a red mini-skirt and looked beautiful - And I felt so happy.

"Hi Davy."

"Hi Bubbles."

"Davy, can you hold the towel in your backpack?"

"Sure."

We rode to the community park. There were people everywhere. We spent a long time looking for Lichuan and Cheryl, but couldn't find them. We laid the towel on the ground.

"Davy, the towel's wet."

"It's your sweat, Bubbles..."

"It's your sweat."

"No way, Bubbles. You were the one who used it today at the pool."

The couple next to us lit some sprinklers, and we watched them wave them in the air.

"I remember when I was home on the Fourth of July," she said. "My parents would spend like fifty dollars on fireworks. We had all kinds of things..."

"Snakes, sprinklers, volcanoes..."

"Yeah, all that."

She broke off suddenly and put her face flat on the towel.

"I miss my family, Davy."

"I'm sorry, Bubbles."

Suddenly, I was gripped by a childhood memory.

"What are you thinking about, David?"

"I was just remembering something. You ever think about how selfish kids are?... I was at the park with my brother and my mom on the Fourth of July. She was lighting a sprinkler, and it blew up in her hand. She was burned and we had to go home."

I hesitated.

"Bubbles, all I could think of was how much I wanted to stay."

I shook my head.

"My poor mother," I sighed.

Bubbles looked on me, quietly...

The fireworks began. We sat watching the dazzling display of lights and colors glow in the sky, and the warmth of her body, sound of her full laughter, and glimpse of her smile as she lay next to me.

Leaving was a problem because everyone left at once and crowded the exits.

We went to The Graduate and shared a Grad-burger. A lot of the people were singing bar songs.

Leaving, we rode our bikes to my lab. The bar songs still in my head, I began to sing.

> *Da dum, Da dum,*
> *Go to the bar,*
> *Da dum, da dum,*
> *Order a beer,*
> *Da dum, da dum,*
> *Get drunk,*
> *Da dum, da dum,*
> *Go home,*
> *Da dum, da dum...*

"Throw up!" Bubbles chimed in with laughter. "You're a good singer, Davy."

"Who's singing?..."

We parked our bikes outside the Chem Building and went inside. I put on a tape and began dancing, Bubbles smiling and laughing all the while.

"Don't stop, David. Dance some more."

I took a Michael Jackson tape out of my desk and played it on the tape recorder.

> *When you feel that beat,*
> *and we can ride the boogie.*
> *Feel that beat of love...*

Sitting on her lap, she uncrossed her legs underneath me and put her arms around my waist.

"Where did you learn to dance, David?"

"I didn't. I just went to parties."

"Can you swing?"

"What's that?"

"I'll show you."

We got up and stood in the middle of the room.

"It's like this," she said.

She took my hands in hers, walked back, turned with a lift of the leg and went back.

I caught on quickly. I had always wanted to dance close with someone, but never felt comfortable with other girls. Now, with Bubbles, it was exactly how I imagined it. She twirled into my arms with no inhibitions.

That was it, I thought. In Bubbles there aren't inhibitions. I feel happy and full of life.

When the song ended I turned off the tape and we walked to the X-ray diffraction lab. I showed Bubbles some crystals under the polarizing microscope. She thought they were beautiful and enjoyed watching me work.

Dancing through the corridors on our way out, Bubbles laughed approvingly.

We rode home and immediately went to bed...

CHAPTER THREE

Monday, July 9, 1984

It's 6:15 PM and I'm sitting in the x-ray diffraction room. Professor Hope is working quietly on the omega scans. I'm very tense. I'd been unsuccessful at determining the unit size for the crystal I've been working on, which is small and imperfectly mounted and has a difficult extinction. Now Professor Hope is making slow progress.

One final concern - I'm supposed to be home at 7 PM to go to San Francisco with Bubbles.

Just before we got started I'd told him I'd tried everything I knew, but nothing seemed good enough.

"You know what is the best thing to do when things like that happen on a Friday afternoon," he said in his thick Norwegian accent. "The best thing to do is take off the crystal and have a good weekend."

Nevertheless, we did go downstairs to the diffractometer to see if anything could be done. There was, and Professor Hope showed me a new strategy for unit cell diffraction.

We were nearly finished with the preliminary study when I noticed that there were some aspects of the work that could be enhanced.

"Professor Hope, are we going to obtain high angle reflections to improve the standard deviations?"

"No," he responded chipperly. "We are going to go home and have dinner."

A few minutes later we were finished. The only thing I could think of was how I couldn't wait to get home and get ready to go to

San Francisco with Bubbles. I arranged with Stuart Riley to turn off the machine tomorrow and left for Bubbles'.

I pedaled into the night. I was feeling happy and excited. I'd been in Davis for two years and still hadn't gone to San Francisco – Priorities like school and research were always in the way.

Going to San Francisco with Bubbles was special. A year ago she and I had been roommates in the same apartment. One day we were waiting in line at the Lucky's Supermarket and talking about the fact that I'd never been to San Francisco.

"You've never been to San Francisco?" the cashier interrupted.

"No, I haven't."

"You've never been to the Wharf?"

"No."

"You've never eaten sour dough and crab meat on the Wharf there?"

"I'm sorry. No, I haven't."

"Oh, my God! You've got to go…"

That day Bubbles and I made three promises to each other - To go to temple, to go to San Francisco, and to go to Venice, Italy…

I got to Bubbles', parked my bike and leapt up the stairs.

"Hi Bubbles."

"Hi Davy. You know what?… Keith called and said he isn't going to be ready to leave until nine."

"Nine! Damn. I left the lab early just so I could be back here ready to go… No, there was nothing left to do in the lab. Bubbles, what are we going to do until nine?"

"You can give me a back massage if you want to."

"Sure."

She laid on the bed, and I began massaging her. Her eyes rolled up as her lids gently closed over them.

"Oh, Davy, you give good back rubs."

Suddenly, her eyes opened wide.

"Davy, you want to give me a body rub?"

"Sure."

I felt uneasy. I wanted to give her a body rub, but I wondered where I could put my hands? And where I couldn't?! To say nothing of where I shouldn't?

I kept massaging her back. Finally, I went to her thighs.

"David, you have to massage my head and neck, too."

Her hair was wonderfully soft. She closed her eyes gently and breathed comfortably.

Bubbles, I thought, I could devote my entire life to giving you pleasure. For you I would give my time, my heart, my life, my love.

I put her hands on my thighs and massaged them. A vacuum was created between our hands.

"David, that feels so good."

I massaged her hips. For reassurance she and I kept talking. She was ticklish when I got to her feet, but that didn't last long.

Facing her now, I massaged her legs. She just smiled, spoke and laughed the whole time.

Bubbles, I thought, don't you know how beautiful you are? In your eyes I see twinkling stars - Outstretched and inviting me to explore them.

When I finished, she looked up and smiled. I was smiling, too. I wanted to kiss her, but couldn't, and instead massaged her hands a little longer, then told her it was her turn to massage me.

"Massage you?!" she exclaimed. "Well, I don't know. I could just lay here all day."

"No, Bubbles. It's my turn."

I laid on the bed and felt her hands in my hair.

"Davy, you have so much hair."

She was massaging my arms when I felt her tugging at my watch.

"No, Bubbles, you can't take my watch off."

"Yes, David... I have to massage your wrists."

"My wrists don't need it."

"Yes, David."

She took off the watch, revealing baby-white skin underneath.

"Wow, I bet I could get you to take off anything," she said. "Everything."

I became ticklish when she massaged my sides and writhed underneath her.

"David, I'm going to stop massaging you if you don't stop moving."

"I can't help it, Bubbles."

"Well, stop it."

"I can't," I managed between bursts of laughter.

Then, she slid her finger nails over my sides, and I involuntarily my arms back and struck her thigh. I heard an anguished giggle, then felt her hair on my back as her head fell forward.

"David!..."

"Sorry, Bubbles."

"You have to kiss it now."

I moved my head to kiss her leg.

"No, David. It's over here."

I moved as much as her straddle hold would let me.

"David, why are you so sensitive?"

"I don't know. I just am."

"Is it because you don't like it when people touch you?"

"It's because I like being touched too much."

"Are you a good lover?"

"The best."

She massaged my face.

"Gee, I can fit three fingers on each side of your nose."

"I wouldn't talk, Bubbles."

She finished by taking my hands and smiling...

At nine we met Keith outside. He had a powerful black truck, and we drove to Concord, where he dropped us off at a gas station. From there Bubbles' sister, Carol, picked us up and drove us to her mobile home.

Bubbles and I were pretty tired; we found a spot on the floor and slept the rest of the night.

We woke up early the next morning. Carol had class in a community college in Orinda, so she dropped Bubbles and I off at the BART station and we took it to the Civic Center in SF. We caught the N bus for Golden Gate Park. Stepping out on the street we saw a policeman on horseback.

"Oh, I want a picture of a mounted policeman," she said.

"I'll take it, Bubbles."

The policeman stayed to take the picture, then smiled and waved and trotted off.

Next we saw a horse-drawn carriage.

"Bubbles, stand next to it and I'll take another picture."

Bubbles coyly walked forward. There was iced champagne in the carriage.

"How much are rides?" she asked the driver.

He was preoccupied with me aiming the camera.

"Smile and take the picture, darling," he said...

"David, let's go to the Japanese Tea Gardens."

"Alright."

I think we both wanted to hold hands, but walked separately.

I paid for tickets and we entered the gardens. I was hungry and bought some fortune cookies. We exchanged fortunes.

"Here's one, Bubbles. 'You will never be hungry.' This one must have been written before I began living in the Chem lab."

"I don't like mine," she said.

"What does it say?"

"'You will attain wealth through marriage.'"

"I wouldn't like that one, either."

Passing a waste basket, she took the fortune out of her pocket, crumpled it up and threw it away.

Walking through the garden, every turn revealed another new and beautiful sight. I would ask Bubbles to stand in front of a pond, and she me next to a Pagoda.

I got up on a steep, high bridge. Just as she was about to snap the picture, she stopped.

"David, I want to take a picture with you."

I called to a woman walking under the bridge.

"Excuse me, Ms. Can you take a picture of us?"

"Sure, but it'll have to be quick. I have to get back to my party."

"Come on up, Bubbles."

She gave the woman the camera and climbed the bridge.

"Is the camera loaded?" called the woman.

"I'll check," I said, leaping from the bridge and running to her. "Yes, it's loaded. Just push the button."

Bubbles and I put our arms around each other, and the woman snapped the picture.

"It looks like the two of you are in the clouds," she said.

Bubbles and I left the Gardens and hadn't walked far before we reached the Arboretum.

"Let's go in there, Bubbles."

"Alright."

Our eyes lit up with excitement; the grounds were lined with a beautiful assortment of plants and greenery. White swans filled the pond. We walked towards them slowly; they didn't fly away, but just parted to form a path for us to follow.

"Bubbles, I love this."

We held hands.

"David, let's sit down on the bench. I always like to sit on park benches and look at the park."

"Okay."

We sat on the bench. I stood up a moment later.

"Let's go," I said.

Bubbles began to get up. I took her hand.

"I'm just kidding, Bubbles. Let's sit for a while."

I crossed my legs and looked out at the park. Bubbles took my hand and rubbed my fingers.

We walked through a row of trees that led to a beautifully lit summit. Then, the ground began to sink underneath us.

"David, do you think the trail is okay?"

I took another step - The ground was solid.

"I think it's okay."

The next step my shoe sank deep into the grass.

"David, it's mud."

"I know."

Bubbles began to laugh.

"I spoke too soon, Bubbles."

We took several more steps - Mud in every direction.

"Bubbles, there can't be much more."

More mud.

"Bubbles, I can't get it right."

She laughed.

Finally we got to the summit. We took more pictures and kept walking.

We wandered to a beautiful lake. It looked like a sight from a tropical paradise novel. Pagodas surrounded it, and above flowed a wall of water.

We thought about renting a paddle boat, but it was getting late and we had to meet Carol at the Wharf.

We were lost now. We wandered through the park holding hands.

We came to a Rose Garden and walked along the rows of flowers, sharing our favorites with each other.

We came out along a dirt road. The sand was fine and wet, and we found ourselves sinking again.

We were sitting on a tree-trunk when I saw a couple approaching.

"Excuse me, sir. We're kind of lost."

"Where do you want to be?"

"The Wharf."

"Whoa. You are pretty lost..."

"We want to go to the Wharf," Bubbles insisted.

He produced a map, and we made a plan.

Bus 28 pulled up and we climbed in. I was about to put two bill in the receptacle.

"No bills," the driver said. "This bus only takes change."

I knew I didn't have any.

"Well, let me look through my wallet," I said.

"You're holding up traffic. If you don't pay by the next stop, you'll have to get off."

The bus pulled out.

"Does anyone in the bus have change?" I cried out. "Is there anyone with change for a dollar?"

An elderly woman came forward and gave us change. She looked poor and her clothes were in tatters - She was the last person I thought would help.

We fell asleep as the bus drove on. I woke up first.

"Bubbles, look. It's the Golden Gate Bridge."

We admired its size and beauty.

The area where we were dropped off was close to the bay and surrounded by boats. I saw a couple walking with their toddler daughter and asked if they'd take a picture? The man directed us towards a background with the most boats; the woman in the direction with the most light.

On the way to the Wharf we stopped to watch the boats, fishermen and look out at the Alcatraz.

The Wharf was crowded and the sidewalks packed with people. We shopped for a good deal on sourdough and crabmeat.

Our crab and sourdough bread in hand, we walked to Pier 39 looking for Carol. When we didn't find her, we took a table and began to eat. The bread melted in our mouths, and we exchanged smiles of pure pleasure. It was much better than I'd anticipated - but, then, I hadn't had any expectations.

We went to a store in Chinatown. I saw a toy bear that jumped rope and couldn't resist getting it for her.

In another store I found some toy swords; Bubbles and I fenced along the aisles, then I turned and knighted all the children who had been giggling as they watched. Before we left the store, she bought the sword for me.

Leaving the store I saw a guitarist and saxophonist on the corner across the street. I gave Bubbles my sword, walked over to the players, deposited a dollar in their hat, then tried break-dancing as a crowd gathered to watch. When I got up, Bubbles stood smiling, then eagerly took me into her arms.

Bubbles wanted to ride the trolley before leaving San Francisco. The last trolley was about to depart from the station, and I took her by the hand and made a running dash. We jumped on the moving car and held on by the rails.

"David, you are so much fun."

I felt her warm lips press against my neck, then cheek.

"I'm so happy to be with you tonight," she said.

We returned to Concord, and Carol picked us up at the station. Inside the mobile home Bubbles and I sat on the couch. She was laying with her head in my lap and playing with Carol's miniature terrier; I gently ran my fingers through her hair...

CHAPTER FOUR

Tuesday, July 10, 1984

It's a little past 10 PM. I'm in the lab with Brendan. Both of us are signed up for the computer all night. I have six or more crystals to refine. I have a deadline posted on them - Tomorrow. Two crystals for Professor Smith, one for Professor Hurt, and four for Professor Poole. Each refinement requires a lot of thinking and even more time. It's going to be a long night.

I had begun reading Stout and Jensen *X-ray crystallography* when suddenly I heard a gentle rapid tap on the window that sent shock waves through my body. Looking, I saw a tall scantly lit figure spastically waving at me.

"Bubbles?"

I ran from the lab to the side entrance to the Chem Building and met her at the door.

"Hi David."

"Hi Bubbles. What are you doing here?"

"I wanted to drop by and see you. Cheryl and I just saw *Ghostbusters.* It was so good. It was great. It was so funny."

Bubbles' face lit up with excitement as she talked. I'd been wanting to see her all day.

"What are you doing right now, David?"

"I'm waiting for the computer to finish a couple of cycles for the refinement of one of my structures. Bubbles, I have so much work. This is going to be another late night."

"Oh, David, I'm sorry..."

"There's nothing to feel bad about. Just a lot of work. It's no big deal."

"What time did you work till last night?"

"About six in the morning..."

"Six!"

"Yeah - You didn't hear me when I came in?... I was pretty noisy."

"No, I was dead last night. I didn't hear anything."

"Well, that's what time I came in. I don't think tonight's going to be any different."

"David, you have to take care of yourself."

"I got to do what I got to do," I mumbled. "So, Bubbles, you want to dance with me downstairs?"

"Will you teach me a new dance?"

"Yes," I said, smiling widely.

I told her to wait downstairs while I started another refinement cycle. When I arrived I saw her sitting at my desk drawing on a scrap of paper. She was penciling a WAAH face and a horse.

"Beautiful, Bubbles. You know what, you should make me a big drawing of a WAAH face."

"Why do you want a big WAAH face?"

"Because I want one. A big one - Like this," I spread my arms open wide.

I put on the Michael Jackson tape and snapped my fingers as I made my way back to her.

"David, how do you spin?"

"Like this."

I put one foot behind the other and spun on my left heel.

Bubbles tried it, but got her legs tangled and she nearly fell. She tried again, but looked as though she were jumping. Both of us laughed.

"Now show me, David."

"Okay, like this."

I did a spin, then she tried.

"That's great, Bubbles."

She spun again and again.

"Don't get yourself dizzy, Bubbles."

She just laughed.

"You know what," I said, "I think I like swinging with you the best."

"Okay."

She took my hands and began to swing; moving close, pushing away with a quarter turn, then close again. She smiled all the time, laughing as she twirled back and forth, and moving me as I curled my arms around her - Singing all the while.

We slow danced to the next song. Holding each other close, she moved her arms up and down my back.

The song that followed was too fast to swing to. As I went to fast forward it. Bubbles sat on the stool.

"You like dancing, don't you, David?"

"Love it."

"Is it you favorite thing to do?"

"No... My second favorite."

"What's your first."

"I'm not sure."

"Dancing is one of your favorite past times, though."

"Definitely," I said moving close to her. "When I'm on the dance floor, I can do whatever I want."

"Can't you always do that?"

"No. Some things I'd like to do, but people would think I was crazy. I'm sorry, Bubbles, I'm just a kid at heart."

"I know. You're so silly."

"Yeah, but you love it."

"I know," she said shaking her head and laughing. "You were so great in San Francisco - Getting out your sword and stopping traffic. I thought you were crazy, but I loved it."

I moved close to her, and massaged her shoulders and gently swung her from side to side. We kept talking; every time she laughed she would press her head to my chest and hold me. Her face lit, she looked beautiful.

"That feels so good, David."

"You know what, I think I know what I like doing most," I said. "I like massaging you more than anything else."

"Oh, I'm going to remember that," she said, laughing, her head to my chest again.

It was getting late and I had to get back to my research and Bubbles to bed. I followed her as she left the building.

It's 6 am now. I've been working on the computer all night. I'm very tired, but the thought of last night makes me smile and fills me with energy...

CHAPTER FIVE

Friday, July 13, 1984

As the days pass I find myself more and more captivated by Bubbles. The feelings between us grow, and my respect for her continues. I do feel love for her, but it is the most unselfish love I have ever experienced. There is no desire to possess her; only a feeling of joy and delight in her company.

On Wednesday she was determined to keep me from spending all night in the Chem lab the way I had the previous two nights. She called and asked if she could study with me? I was delighted.

Just before she arrived, though, I had a confrontation with Professor Hope. He said he knew I was working hard, but he wasn't impressed; I had taken on more than I could handle and lost my purpose.

Although he meant well, I felt rejected and humiliated.

I went outside to wait for Bubbles. The thought of my poor performance burned in my head. I lay down on the ground.

Then, I heard the clanking of a bicycle in the distance.

"You better move," Bubbles said. "I'm going to run over you."

I lay there. She locked her bike and came over.

"What's the matter, David?"

"I just got a talking to by Professor Hope."

She sat next to me.

"He says I'm taking on too much and comprehending too little."

"Doing too much at one time isn't good," she said. "I remember when..."

Her words became a blur. All I knew was that her consolation was removing the anger I directed against myself.

She got up, and reaching out my hand, she lifted me. We walked hand-in-hand into the building.

I escorted her to the lab to study while I worked on the computer.

When I came back, she was sitting at the desk, smiling.

"How are you doing, Bubbles?"

"Fine. Hey, you know what?... A little man came and visited me."

"A little man?!... Oh, no - Professor Hope?!"

"Yeah. He's a nice man."

"What did he say?"

"We just talked for a little while. He asked me if I was David's friend who goes to temple with him, and I said yes."

"You're kidding..."

"Yeah. He said he wanted to talk to you. I told him you were around somewhere."

"What else did he say?"

"He told me something about you, too."

I walked towards her.

"What?"

I sat on her lap. She put her arms around me.

"I can't tell you... It's personal."

"Bubbles..."

"I'm just teasing, Davy. He didn't say anything about you. He said I should take you home and put you to bed. I told him I was trying."

I began to laugh.

"He looks like a man who really loves life. I can see why you like him."

While she studied, I cooked quesadillas on the portable electric stove. We danced after we ate; holding each other close, talking, laughing. I had my arms around her waist while she slowly massaged my chest.

She refused to leave unless I left with her; it was nothing forceful - She just said she wanted to stay in the lab as long as I did.

At 1 am I finished my computer runs and told her it was time to go.

We sang along the way. She asked if I'd like to go with her to the side-walk sale tomorrow? I said I'd love to.

We walked hand-in-hand at the sale. She took me from place to place, asking what I thought of the shorts, shoes and panties she picked out?

I couldn't resist getting her some flowers at one of the stands we passed. I got her a long, wide stemmed flower with orange petals, with some still yet to bloom.

We met Professor Hope just before we were going back. He was with a woman named Mindy. I had a camera and took a picture of he, Mindy and Bubbles.

"I'll call it 'Professor Hope and the ladies'," I told Bubbles.

"You mean 'The ladies and Professor Hope'," she responded...

Later that evening Bubbles came to the lab to study with me. A song by Earth Wind and Fire came on the radio and we began to dance. She jokingly rubbed her face against my unshaven cheek. I told her she was going to get a rash. She laughed and said it reminded her of when she was a little girl and her father would ask her for a kiss, then rub his rough, unshaven beard against her until it would become red.

She stared at me.

"You're very handsome, David," she said suddenly. I was embarrassed. "Especially when you smile."

We continued to slow dance, talking and laughing in each other's arms.

"I really like you, David."

"I love you, Bubbles." The words just flowed out; it happened naturally.

She looked at me as I held her.

"I really like this, David. This is much better than last summer."

"I like this, too, Bubbles. Last summer was great, too. Coming home and cooking. Making fish and then Mexican dinners. It was great..."

"But we were studying all the time. Now - Well, we're working, but we have more time together."

"I know. I'm really enjoying it."

"I must really be a distraction to you."

"You?... How about me to you?"

"Well, you hardly got any work done tonight or last night."

"I got a lot done last night..."

"You did?"

"Yes... But, Bubbles, I got to tell you, the time I spend with you is just as if not more important than the time I spend doing research this summer." I hesitated. "You're very, very special, Bubbles."

"You are, too, David."

We left for home. When we walked out of the building, Bubbles asked me for a hug. I asked if I could kiss her. We walked our bikes home and sang along the way.

We got ready for bed. It had been two weeks of me living with her, I thought; sooner-or-later one of her dorm-mates was bound to want me thrown out. I would miss Bubbles when that day came.

Bubbles entered the room.

"David, if you like I'll give you a back massage."

I smiled, got up off the floor and laid on the bed. Her fingers moved over my shoulders and back. When she got to my sides, I thought, 'Don't resist, Dave. Just let your love flow out.' I didn't squirm this time, but breathed deep and enjoyed it.

After a long time I turned over and told her it was her turn.

I ran my fingers through her hair.

"My hair is so thin..."

"So soft," I countered.

"It's not thick like yours."

"It's beautiful."

Moving down her body, when I finished at her feet, she grasped my fingers with her toes and held them there, laughing and smiling.

I told her to turn over.

"Wow!" she said.

I turned off the light to help her rest, then continued to massage her. Her eyes closed, arms above her head, she looked relaxed.

I wondered how she was feeling about my massaging her? If she was uncomfortable? She breathed out a gentle sigh.

"I love your touch," she said.

We were both relaxed. She licked her lips.

When I finished, I kissed her, then got down off the bed and laid on the floor.

She got up and left the room. When she returned, she gazed out the window.

"Isn't the sky beautiful tonight?" she said.

I got up and stood at the window next to her. The sky was lit with stars.

"Yes, it's beautiful," I said.

We went back to our respective covers.

"Thank you for the massage, David," she said.

"I enjoy massaging you, Bubbles."

She laughed.

"You shouldn't say that. You don't know what you're getting yourself into. Goodnight, David..."

CHAPTER SIX

Sunday, July 15, 1984

The days pass and the endearment between Bubbles and I grows.

Friday night we went to temple. The building was packed. The rabbi was on vacation, and one of the young female congregants led the service.

After, we munched on desserts. Bubbles enjoyed the small chocolate pastries. I said that Jewish pastries were the best, and Chinese pastries couldn't compare.

On the way home Bubbles took me through a tour of the park. Just as we were leaving we got caught in the sprinklers. Both of us laughed the whole time we were riding.

I would have liked to take her for ice cream, but she was taking the GRE the next day, so I decided to save it for another time.

We went to the lab for a couple dances. Just as I turned on the radio and started dancing, one of the post-docs walked in.

"Hi Madelyn," I said.

"Hi," she responded curtly.

She went to her desk, took something out of a drawer, then left without a word.

"Oh, my God," I said. "Bubbles, I'm so embarrassed."

She just shrugged her shoulders.

I still felt embarrassed and worried that Madelyn might come in again, but turned on the radio again and we began to dance.

> *Living crazy, that's the only way.*
> *So tonight, gotta put the 9 to 5 up on the shelf,*

And just enjoy yourself...

"Enjoy yourself, David."

"I am enjoying myself..."

"Always!"

We slow danced; she was close to me, and as we spoke, I got her hair in my mouth.

"I like you, David!" she said.

We danced a little longer, then went back to her dorm. We talked for a while, then went to sleep.

Saturday morning Bubbles took the GRE, and I went to the Chem Building to work on refining a nitro-compound for Professor Hurt.

At 1 PM we met at the Rec Pool and swam, then sat in the sun.

We met Stan and Cheryl there. Bubbles took off with Stan for a movie; Cheryl invited me to her place for dinner.

Cheryl showed me around her apartment, then put on some Adam Ant music while we prepared dinner.

"Dave, you know what? Every time I hear Adam Ant, I think of you."

"He's my favorite."

We cooked chicken. It was the best dinner I'd had since returning to Davis.

After dinner Bubbles and Stan joined us, and we made plans for a party. Bubbles and I went to the market and picked up tortillas and cheese, and Coca Cola for mixing Bacardi.

Sitting at the table playing quarters, Bubbles kept hitting on me.

"David, I'm gonna get you so drunk," she'd say as the quarter fell into the glass, then pushing her elbow into my stomach before sliding the glass in my direction. "You're gonna be wasted..."

Afterwards, Bubbles and I went to the Chem lab for some dancing. We sang *Follow the Yellow Brick Road* as we walked through the corridors.

We'd been dancing for a while when Bubbles stopped to get a drink of water. I sat on the chair next to the radio. Bubbles came over and sat on my lap. I put my arms around her; she put one hand on my chest, and massaged my shoulder with the other. We talked - About the people at the party, how I explained things like a professor, and would make a good instructor one day.

We went back to her place and got washed and ready for bed.

She put on an Eddie Murphy comedy album, and we lay on the bed laughing at nearly every line.

I began massaging her. Her eyes showed how comfortable she was. I was massaging her chest, my hands under her shirt, and I could feel her full breasts.

No, I thought, this isn't a dare; I don't want to chance not massaging her by going too far.

Massaging her face, I gently moved her head from side-to-side. Her wild soft black hair, slender nose, high cheek bones and round, big, beautiful eyes – She was beautiful.

"I'm finished," I said.

Her face broke into a radiant smile.

"Thank you, David."

"Thank you, Bubbles..."

CHAPTER SEVEN

Monday, July 16, 1984

Sunday morning we woke up late.

Bubbles went downstairs to the DC [Dining Commons] and brought me back something to eat.

"Wow, onion! Thank you, Bubbles. I love these bagels."

Eating them, I got cream cheese on my face.

"David, you're such a slob."

After she cleaned the cream cheese from my face, I licked it from her fingers.

Bubbles took me by the hand and began swing dancing to the music of Heuy Lewis on the radio.

"I think it works better in your lab," she said. "David, I like you..."

We left for the Rec Hall and played volleyball. She was impressed at how well I played - I was impressed myself. We began laughing as the shots got crazy, and we had to run all over the waxed wooden floors to get to the ball.

We traded the volleyball for a basketball and went downstairs to the courts. Bubbles was all over me every time I had the ball, and in the end I lost.

When Bubbles made the final shot, I ran to her and told her "Good game" and gave her a big hug.

"You're not mad that I beat you, Davy?"

"No."

She began laughing.

"What are you laughing about, Bubbles?"

"The way you answer questions - 'No' 'Yes' 'Good'. You're so funny."

We lifted weights, then I left the Rec Hall to go to the store, then the lab.

The X-ray diffractometer wasn't in use, so I decided to mount a crystal. There were several complications, and I carefully noted them in the log.

I'd been studying the crystal when Bubbles came that evening. We made tortillas with butter, cheese, scallions and avocado. While I cooked Bubbles made a big "WAAH" poster. I really liked it, and told her I was going to hang it up as soon as she was done.

I turned on the radio and we began to dance. Every time I spun her, she'd finish smiling and laughing.

The song *Could it be I'm Falling in Love* came on, and I sang as we danced.

> *Ever since I met you,*
> *I've begun to feel so strange.*
> *Every time I hear your name –*
> *That's funny...*

"I never heard that line before," she said, as I squinted my eyes to the lyrics of the last line. "David, you make so many expressions - Your eyebrows, the way you move them."

Reaching for a high note, my voice cracked.

"David, we were so cruel to you last summer. Whenever you would sing, me and Tim would always cut you down - 'Oh, Dave's singing again.' 'I think he'd make a good tenor.' 'Yeah, a good tenor-twelve miles away from here.'"

"And now you have to dance with me," I said, "and listen to me sing all the time."

"No, you have a beautiful voice, David - It's just when you try to sing the high notes."

I lifted my head in laughter.

"Bubbles, I love being with you."

"No. I'm a witch, David."

"No way..."

"How do you know?"

"I know."

I moved to kiss her. I saw her eyes close, as she tilted her head. She looked beautiful - Like a dream. I felt the tenderness of her lips on mine. I could have kissed her forever.

We held each and slow danced to the music on the radio.

"When I go home, you're going to be bummed," she said.

"I know."

"You're not going to have anywhere to sleep."

"Bubbles, I don't care where I sleep - I can sleep anywhere. It's you I'll miss."

I kissed her neck.

"Davy," she said looking at me excitedly, "I'll probably come back after two weeks."

"Good."

She started laughing.

"'Good.' David, the way you say that..."

"And then you can come back and live with me in my lab..."

"And get bitten by the rats. No, I think I'm going to live in the sorority."

I let her go.

"Bubbles, when you do come back, you will come and dance with me?"

"Well..."

"Well, maybe..."

"Yes, I will."

"We'll go to the 'in place' in Davis..."

"The 'in place'?..."

"My lab..."

"This is it!"

Another song came on the radio, and we began to swing dance. It was getting late.

"David, we better go back, or I won't be able to get up tomorrow."

"Okay, but can I have a kiss first?"

Her eyes closed, she pressed her lips against mine, and we held each other for a long time.

"Bubbles, I could dance with you forever."

I could feel my heart melt.

We left the lab, and went to the X-ray room to check the crystal. Things were fine; I explained the machinery to her, and she massaged my shoulders as I spoke, and looked at me full of admiration.

At her place I got washed and ready for bed, then massaged her.

"David," she said dreamily, "you have magic hands."

When I finished, I held her hands.

"Buenos noches, senorita muy bonita."

"Goodnight, David..."

CHAPTER EIGHT

Tuesday, July 17, 1984

I woke up early to the sight of Bubbles coming into the room. Wearing the rainbow-dotted undies we'd picked out and tip-toeing from one spot to another so not to wake me, I couldn't help but think this was going to be a wonderful day.

I got up a little later and went to the lab. I discovered that the data collection from the night before had a problem. Madelyn had read my detailed log and found the axial photos questionable. We took another photo and found unwanted reflections. Removing the crystal and examining it under the polarizing microscope, we discovered it was cracked. I was disappointed, but learned a lot.

I spent the rest of the day refining structures with Professor Hope. After, Bubbles and I decided to play tennis. She met me at the lab, and we rode to the courts. I had never played better. I was hitting everything that came over the net, and was literally flying across the court - I must have looked like a dog jumping for a Frisbee.

As Bubbles and I picked up balls at the net, she looked at me and smiled.

"I really like this, David. This is fun."

She turned around and headed back to the far court.

"Bubbles," I called to her. "Come here a minute."

I reached my hands over the net - my racket behind her, and my arms around her waist.

"I'm really enjoying this, too, Bubbles."

"I didn't think I was going to like this, but it's really fun. You're really good, David."

"Bubbles, you're great. I'm really impressed."

"You're just saying that because you like me."

"That, too, but you're really good."

Suddenly, a dream-like look came over her features, and she gently kissed my lips. I was stunned and could feel my heart melt underneath me.

We began to play again. I thought that I wouldn't play as well after what happened, but, if anything, I played even better - Going for the ball - Running fast and free.

When we were ready to leave, Bubbles was still saying how much fun she had and how we had to play again and again.

Bubbles went back to her place, and I returned to the lab. I had to work on refining one of Professor Hurt's structures.

I went to the store to pick up some food; I wanted to get some Ruffles potato chips for Bubbles. Then, suddenly, on the ride back to the lab, I was struck by the thought of what I'd say to her should our relationship ever become something more.

"You don't understand," I told her in my head. "My life has always been geared towards a purpose - some meaning. I can't live my life around one person. I haven't worked this hard to devote my life to loving one person. My life is dedicated to research and the pursuit of applying my knowledge to the greater good..."

I had Bubbles now to cherish and be thankful. When the day comes for her go, I will always have the memories of the time and love we shared this day.

When I arrived at Bubbles', she had just gotten out of the shower and was wearing her undies.

I gave her the Ruffles (They were her favorite), and we shared them until they were nearly all gone.

We studied her GRE booklets till it was time to go to bed.

I got on the bed to massage her.

"David, do you really like doing this?"

"Yes. Do your really like getting it?"

"Yes. I'll never refuse."

I was massaging her hands when she closed them around my fingers and held them tight.

"I'm going to make you my slave, David." I was quiet. "I'm going to put you in chains."

"You don't have to, Bubbles..."

"Then I'm going to whip you - I'm into bondage."

I massaged her legs; she had just shaved them, and they were soft. When I got to her feet, she became ticklish; I continued until she got used to it.

Massaging her waist she became sensitive again.

"David, you're tickling me."

"I'm just feeling you with my fingertips."

"I'm tingling all over."

I stopped and used my whole hands.

"I know I like it. I just don't want to die laughing."

I was massaging her neck when I felt her hands reaching out in the darkness and tenderly massaged my legs, sides and chest. I became immersed in the feeling.

"You're slowing down, David. I'm going to have to stop massaging you." She lowered her hands. "Aren't I selfish?"

"No, Bubbles."

"Yes I am."

"You're the most unselfish person I know."

"You don't know me very well. I'm selfish."

I continued massaging her.

"David, I bet this could be a cure to everything - Headaches, backaches, bellyaches, soreness - Everything."

I could feel her drifting as I massaged her face.

"David," she said with a sigh, "I love your caress."

I was finished, but I didn't want it to end. I ran my hands down her body to her legs again.

"Bubbles, your legs are so soft."

"I know. I should shave them more often..."

"I was just going to say I have to take advantage of this."

"David, you're going to spoil me."

I didn't say anything.

"You know you will."

"Maybe," I said after thinking for a moment, "but right now you feel so good I don't care."

I massaged her abdomen and side again. This time she smiled, but didn't laugh.

"Thought I'd be ticklish, didn't you?"

"Yep," I said. "But I know you're still tingling."

"How do you know?"

"I just know."

"Well," she said and paused, "you're right."

I held her hands and told her goodnight. Her face smiled back at me.

I got off the bed and under my covers on the floor. My fingertips warm and tingling, I felt good inside...

CHAPTER NINE

Wednesday, July 18, 1984

At about 4 PM I was working in Professor Poole's lab. I was making publication tables for Professor Hurt's nitro-Diels Alder structure. Suddenly, I felt someone press a finger into my side.

I turned expecting to see Bob - To my surprise, he spoke with Bubbles' voice.

"Hi David."

It was Bubbles. She was wearing her green, low cut shorts and a loose fitting red-and-white football jersey.

"I had nothing to do, so I thought I'd come by and see what you were doing."

"Don't you have to work?"

"Yes, but I was so tired I decided to take the day off."

I smiled. I was happy she came.

She looked down at my desk.

"What are you doing, David?"

"Putting together some publication tables for Professor Hurt."

"Do you have a lot of work?"

"There's always something to do, Bubbles."

Her look became more thoughtful.

I smiled and got up from my chair.

"Come on, Bubbles. Let's go."

"Where?"

"Out of here."

We left the building through the side entrance.

There was a bandage on her arm.

"Bubbles, how did that happen?"

"A lady grabbed me and stuck a needle in my arm..."

"Bubbles!..."

"Okay, I'll tell you. A giant mosquito came out of the sky and attacked me."

"Bubbles, your nose is growing."

"Maybe it will get as big as yours."

"Hah, hah. Now, what happened?"

"They were taking blood donations at Freeborn Hall and I volunteered."

Something touched me inside.

"That was very nice of you, Bubbles."

I put my arms around her; she put hers around my waist.

"I wouldn't have done it if I had it to do over again."

"Why's that?"

"Because they told me tonight I can't do any running or exercising, and I was planning on lifting weights. I think I'm still going to."

"No way, Bubbles. You'll fall down and die."

"No, I won't. I have an idea. How about if we play tennis tonight?"

"Bubbles, you've got to take it easy."

"I need my daily workout."

"Bubbles..."

"I'll stop if I get tired."

I hesitated and looked down. I didn't want her to, but at least this way I could watch her.

"Alright, Bubbles. What time do you want to go?"

"Anytime. When can you go?"

"Anytime."

"How about when it gets a little warmer..."

"Warmer?..."

She laughed.

"I mean cooler - Seven."

"Sounds good," I said. "So you decided to take the day off. You're going to have to tell me next time - I'll get tickets for us to take the Berkeley bus."

"You really like San Francisco."

"Loved it. We got to go back there again."

"I remember when I used to hate going to San Francisco. Now I can spend days there."

She looked around.

"David, let's walk."

We started towards Stoney Lake and held hands.

"I remember the first time I gave blood," I said. "It was terrible. I was the Vice-President for this honor society called Knights and Ladies; I had arranged the blood drive, so I was the first to give. There were some guys around me saying stuff like 'Don't get nervous, Dave' and 'Here comes the needle.' I got so nervous - When the woman stuck me, I felt this hot splash on my face and heard the others scream - 'Gusher'. I got blood on my face, my shirt, the woman's dress - Made all the people around me sick..."

"I could just see them all gagging."

"Yeah, and they had to give next."

We laughed.

Stoney Lake was in front of us. There were ducks and geese all along the pond.

"Bubbles, this reminds me of a hotel where my relatives used to come to stay when they visited us in California. It had a duck pond - like this, but much smaller.. There were all these ducks, and I always wanted one. I almost got one. My uncle made me let it go."

"How old were you?"

"I must have been ten." I reflected. "I had it. As a matter of fact, it was a goose I had. Yeah, I had it - I'm glad, though, that my uncle made me let it go."

We walked along the creek, then through the rose gardens in the horticulture area. We watched the slowly rippling water; I felt very happy to be with her.

We went back to the lab. We began talking about organic chemistry. I told her how much I enjoyed it; it was fun for me because I could look at the mechanisms like a lot of bumper cars crashing into each other and forming new molecules.

Then, I found myself kissing her between sentences. It was so natural it didn't even interrupt the flow of our conversation.

It came time for Bubbles to go home and study for a while. I went back to my lab.

At about 7 PM I saw Bubbles sitting outside the Chem Building.

"Hello pretty lady."

"Hello guy."

"Can I invite you into my lab?"

"I don't know. It might be dangerous."

"Yeah, with all that exploding ether and all," I said, trying to downplay things.

We went to Professor Poole's lab so I could get my tennis racket. The radio was on, and the song *Footloose* was playing, and Bubbles began moving her feet. I watched her, then got up and took her hand.

"Come on, Bubbles."

We ran downstairs to the other lab. I turned on the radio.

"Let's dance, Bubbles."

"I was dancing," she said, frowning.

"Oh, I'm sorry. I wanted you to dance with me."

We began swing dancing, and I twirled her until the light came back to her face.

We left to play tennis. Bubbles was moving all the time - Running when she collected balls; doing jumping jacks when she had to wait.

Afterwards, she went home to study, and I returned to the lab.

I met one of the graduate students, Stuart Riley, in the X-ray diffraction room. His crystals were beautiful, but something was wrong and he wasn't having any success at determining their unit cell and space group.

I stayed and helped him. We waited a long time for the computer to make its calculations.

"I hate this," he said.

"I know," I responded. "I can feel my heartbeat racing."

Stuart laughed.

A solution came out. The unit cell was orthorhombic and the dimensions were determined.

I left at about eleven to go home. I thought I'd learned a lot by staying.

When I arrived at Bubbles', the door was open but the lights were out.

I quietly crept inside and went to the side of the bed where Bubbles was. She turned over on her back.

"Hi David," she said wearily.

"Hi Bubbles," I whispered. "When did you get to bed?"

She looked at the clock.

"About an hour and a half ago - I'm a bum, I know. I like to sleep."

I smiled.

"What were you doing, David?"

"I was helping a graduate student put on a crystal."

She let out a sigh and stretched her arms.

"Bubbles, can I give you a body massage?"

"'Can you?...'"

"Yes."

"David, do you really like giving me body massages."

I hesitated and looked down. Then I looked at her seriously.

"Bubbles, can I tell you something?"

"Yes."

"Before leaving to come back to Davis, I spent a lot of time with my friend, Ben. The last time we talked he told me that his favorite part of making love to his girlfriend was the happiness it gave her. He said the greatest gift was to give another person pleasure. Bubbles, that's the way I feel when I massage you."

"Do you really want to massage me?"

"Very much."

She turned, and I massaged her.

She was wearing a bikini bottom. Taking in her whole back it dawned on me what a beautiful woman she was.

I was careful with her calves, thinking they were probably sore from the tennis. Again, she was ticklish at her toes, but got used to it.

I enjoyed rubbing her thighs. They were soft and relaxed, and I could literally mold the shape of my hands into them.

I gently ran my fingertips under her night-shirt. I was surprised that she wasn't sensitive this time. In the darkness her teeth and eyes glimmered as she smiled at me.

I gently massaged around her chest, careful not to go too far.

When my hands reached hers, she ran hers over mine with her fingertips. I felt as though in a dream, weightlessness as our hands caressed. I poignant feeling crept into my chest. I closed my eyes and breathed deep.

As I moved my hands to her shoulder and neck, she ran her fingertips along my legs.

I moved to massaged her face. Bending low my lips caressed hers and we kissed.

I moved my hand to her breasts; I felt their gentle outlines as I circled them. She put her hand over mine and guided me.

I was surprised how soft they were; I expected them to be firm, but instead felt like bubbles of air under my fingers.

Her hands in my hair, rubbing my scalp approvingly and keeping my lips close to her body.

Then, she turned my head and kissed my earlobes; I could feel her breath and tingled all over.

Taking off her undies, they were moist.

I reached down to unzip my shorts.

"David," she said softly in the darkness.

"Yes," I said.

"I'm afraid to make love to you."

I raised my head, and looked up at her - I was afraid, too.

"That's okay," I said.

"I want to make love to you, David, but I'm afraid."

"It's okay, Bubbles. I don't need to make love to you. All I need is your smile - your laugh - To dance with you."

"You're very special, David."

"No. You're special." I was fully awake now. "I remember in the dorms last year - We all owed Tanya money for something, and she wrote our names on the boards, and the only two with check marks for having paid were yours and Mary's. I just thought to myself, 'It figures. Bubbles and Mary - the two angels.'"

"I like Mary,"

I hesitated, then kissed her. She put her hand to my lips, and I kissed her fingers.

"Bubbles, you touch a part of me I thought was closed off to others. I love you so much."

"I love you, too, David."

"I remember the first time you said that to me, Bubbles. It was after Professor Hope got so angry at me. I felt so bad - So mad at myself. And, then, you pulled me over to you - Told me you were worried about me - Showed how much you cared. Bubbles, that meant everything to me."

"I care about you so much, David."

She ran her fingers through my hair.

"I love you very much."

I picked up my shorts, and Bubbles put on her undies and went to the bathroom. I left the room, too.

Returning, I stood at the door, feeling confused.

Inside, I could see Bubbles' outlines in the darkness, sitting up in the bed.

"David, would you sleep with me tonight?"

I felt touched.

"Yes," I said.

I got into the bed and under the covers. Bubbles moved close to me and put her head on my shoulder, cuddling me and putting her hand on my chest.

I ran my fingers along her shoulder. Feeling her breath on my chest, drifting off to sleep, I felt so happy...

CHAPTER TEN

Thursday, July 19, 1984

I woke up early the next morning. Bubbles was still curled up next to me. I ran my fingers through her tangled hair, brushing it out of her eyes. Awakening, she licked her lips, and when I ran my fingertips across her face she kissed my hand.

I got up and took a shower in the guys' bathroom. When I came back, Bubbles was dressed and about to leave. She looked fresh, beautiful and happy.

She gave me a hug and wished me a good day.

Could Bubbles really be so happy? I wondered. Had I gone too far? Had I taken advantage of her generous and giving nature? It would make me feel so bad if when I came home today she didn't want me to give her a massage because she felt she couldn't trust me.

I called her at 5 PM - No answer.

Again at six - This time she was home, and we talked for a long time. The enthusiasm in her voice again surprised me. She told me that she'd fallen asleep in class, and her day in radiology was boring because there were so few pet patients; tonight she was going to a movie with Dan. I was happy to hear her voice, but still there were the questions.

I came home late. As usual, the door was wide open and waiting for me. Bubbles was on the bed talking on the telephone, and acknowledged my presence with a twinkle in her eyes.

I sat down on the end of the bed. She extended her arms to me, and massaged my back, shoulders and neck; I felt the sensation of my chest caving for the eruption of sadness and worry that I'd carried all day.

I got up and washed. When I came back, she was lying on the bed with the lights and radio on.

I sat beside her. My lips were dry, and I reached out with my hands to massage her neck.

Looking into her eyes I wondered how she felt? From a gut level I felt things were alright between us, as she relaxed under my touch.

She looked at me and smiled and tilted her head.

"David, it looks like your searching."

"I'm always searching."

"Always?"

As I ran my fingertips along her face, her hands massaged me. Then, with her hands in my hair, she pulled me towards hers. Our noses touched, and I kissed her. I could feel her arms tighten around me, and she let out a happy sigh. I felt the smoothness of her glittering teeth, and she bit on my lower lip. Then, she reached out her arms and held my head tight; then, kissed me – Full and moist.

With a light, persistent pressure she directed me down her body. I kissed the outlines of her breasts; her hands moved through my hair and pushed my lips down harder.

She spoke softly.

"David, I want to make love to you."

The words seized my heart.

"Are you sure, Bubbles?"

"Positive."

I unzipped my shorts, then took off her undies. I wasn't ready, though. Bubbles spoke into my ear again.

"David. I don't have protection , so you can't cum in me."

I continued to rub, but was too nervous. I felt inside her; the warm fluids felt good on my fingers.

I thought that, perhaps, if I massaged her it would stimulate me. As I did, I felt her hand around me; but still I couldn't get hard.

I got up to go to the bathroom.

"I'll be right back, Bubbles."

I kissed her hands; then, turning, felt them still holding me there in my mind. I looked back; she was lying still in the bed.

"David," she said. "Hold me."

Tears welled up in my eyes. I went back and kissed her.

Bubbles left the room. When she returned, she turned out the lights and stopped in the center of the room. I got up and stood naked before her. Excited, I stroked her breasts. She just smiled...

"David, I enjoy loving you," she said afterwards.

She laid on top of me, then lifted her head so I couldn't reach her lips.

She turned to one side and my fingernail caught her.

"Oh, I'm sorry, Bubbles."

I kissed her over and over.

"If this is what I get for being scratched, you're going to have to do it more often."

At about 7 am I decided to go to my lab. I got out of bed.

"Are you leaving me?" she asked.

I turned.

"Not when you put it that way," I said.

I went back. She aroused me with burning kisses along my neck.

Finally I turned to go; Bubbles wishing me a good day...

CHAPTER ELEVEN

Saturday, July 21, 1984

The days pass and I am more attached to Bubbles, while still maintaining my hard work. Every moment that I'm with her, I want to hold her, kiss her. I come back from the lab for a couple of hours of rest; I go to Bubbles' with a flower; at first she scolds me for getting her presents; then takes it; holds me tight; tells me that I'm a sweetheart.

Holding her hand I sat on the bed and pull her close to me.

Bubbles gets up and says she wants some Ruffles. She gets the bag, opens it, and comes back. She puts one chip in her mouth, then one into mine. She laughs as I consume the large chips without using my hands.

Finally, it's time for us to go. Bubbles has her Kaplan course, and I returned to the lab. There is a great deal of work to be done. It consumes - or rather - I am consumed by it. I'm exhausted yet I continue to push. I am not learning so much now as working and achieving, and I can't help but fear that one of the provisions of my life that I always thought would come true is on its way to happening - I cannot share my life without sacrificing my work. The thought horrifies me - lifelong loneliness. I have to find a way to have both...

CHAPTER TWELVE

Sunday, July 22, 1984

The night before I had come home exhausted to find Bubbles wasn't there.

I went to the lounge and laid down on the couch; but sleep wouldn't come - There were too many questions. I hadn't held her in two days. Our separate commitments had kept us apart.

Finally, I became so worried I called an RA and told her I had reason to suspect Bubbles was in trouble because her bike was there and I knew she had a heart condition.

The RA came and opened the door. I was relieved to find that Bubbles wasn't there.

"Thank God," I said.

We found a note on the bed.

> *David,*
> *See ya later,*
> *When? I don't know,*
> *Bubbs*

The RA looked at me confused.

"But if the door was locked, how were you supposed to get the note?"

I laughed.

"Beats the hell out of me..."

The next morning Bubbles found out what happened.

"David, I feel so bad..."

"It's okay, Bubbles. It's okay."

She left for a trip to Marineland. I went to my lab and spent the day working on non-extinguishing crystals - a considerably difficult task. I started at 8 am; by 8 PM I was tired, hungry and exhausted, but something inside drove me to keep on.

I came home to find that Bubbles wasn't there. In the bed my mind was filled with apprehensions. Where is she? I miss her. I miss holding her. I miss loving her.

I lay there for hours; trying to sleep, but not able.

Finally, I heard some rustling in the bathroom, then the knob turning.

"Hi Bubbles," I whispered.

"Hi David."

She sat beside me on the bed and told me about her day. Marineland had not gone as well as she'd anticipated. I felt bad for her; I knew how much she was looking forward to it. I sat up in the bed and stroked her face and kissed her forehead.

We talked more about where she went, her long walk, the wind outside.

She undressed and got into bed with me. She curled up next to me and I kissed her and caressed her back with my fingertips until she was asleep.

I was awoken a little later by the sound of her rubbing her eyes. I sat up and stroked her hair.

"David," she whispered, "I feel so bad. I've felt bad all day. I'm so sorry I locked you out. I'm so stupid. I must have locked the door when I went back for my coat. I'm sorry - I'm so bad!"

I kissed her.

"Bubbles, it's okay. I was just glad you were alright because I was worried about you. You're too hard on yourself - I think you're wonderful; you're the most unselfish and caring person I've ever met."

"I don't see how you think that."

"Your actions say that, Bubbles. Look at you - You go to the movies with Stan because you don't want him to be alone - because you're afraid he's lonely and you know you'd be lonely if you were him. You feel bad because you didn't have a place for me to stay one night, when if it weren't for you and your caring I wouldn't have any place to sleep at all."

"I didn't think of those things."

"Once in a while we just need someone to remind us how wonderful people we are."

She reached out her arms and embraced me, holding me and kissing me. Then, she cuddled to me and went to sleep.

In the morning I woke up to the light of the rising sun. I love the sunrise. During the spring quarter it doesn't matter what time I get to bed - I'll always wake up with the sunrise.

I gently massaged Bubbles' back until she awoke.

"Good morning," she said wearily.

Her sleepy eyes struck me with joy.

"Good morning, Bubbles."

Moving together, inspired by her sighs, I kissed her tenderly...

She lay there after, eyes closed; then raised my head and looked at me.

"David, you're so tender and sincere and loving."

We got up and showered and got ready for the day.

I needed to get some food for the lab and told her I was going to the store.

"Can I go with you, David?"

We walked to the store, singing whatever tunes came into our heads. It didn't matter what the song was - just as long as we knew some of the words. Every now and then I would dance.

"David, you're so silly. I love you."

I felt her hand moving up and down my back.

When we got to my lab, we put the food away and (since Madelyn was there) took a walk to Stoney Lake.

Being with her, everything looked beautiful. We sat on the shore next to the creek and watched the ducks and geese swim by.

We went back to the lab to get a towel and decided to lay out on a patch of grass in front of the Chem Building, so that I could get to the computer between refinement cycles.

I laid the towel on the grass; it had the picture of the moon.

"Think I can take half a moon?" she asked.

Holding her in my arms, I gently pulled her to the center and told her she could have as much as she wanted.

The warmth of the sun, the warmth of her skin, the warmth of her love.

Her eyes closed, I began to sing.

> *Pretty smile on her face,*
> *and I need you tender lady...*

Afterwards I silently watched her.

"I heard you singing, David."

I sang another Chicago song.

> *When I touch you-ou-ou,*

I feel a thousand different feelings...

CHAPTER THIRTEEN

Tuesday, July 31, 1984

Today, Bubbles left on a plane for home.

I told her that she always had my love, but I needed my time to devote to my studies, my research and my pursuit of a career in medicine.

My friend Bob drove Bubbles and I to the airport. I took her bags and started to the counter, while Bob waited.

"I love you, Bubbles. I love you so much. I'll love you forever - Forever and a day."

"I'll love you forever, too, David. I'm so glad you came back this summer. You've made this the best summer I've ever had. I love you."

She walked me back to Bob's car.

"Are we ready to go?" Bob said.

"Yeah."

I kissed her and watched her turn and walk back into the airport terminal.

I opened the door - But was seized with anguish.

"I've got to kiss her one more time," I said.

I went sprinting over.

"Bubbles," I cried.

I ran into her open arms.

"Coming back to me?" she said.

"I love you. I love you so much."

"I love you, David."

I kissed her and held her tight.

I turned and ran back to the car. I closed the door, and Bubbles and I waved to each other as the car drove off.

Now I sit alone, remembering the moments we shared...

CHAPTER FOURTEEN

Last Tuesday Bubbles and I spent a beautiful day at UC Berkeley.

The day before I had made arrangements with Professor Poole to go to Berkeley to deliver some chemical compounds for analysis at the lab of Professor Anderson. I told him I would go on one condition - I wanted Bubbles to go with me. Professor Poole got us the tickets.

That Tuesday Bubbles and I awoke up to the morning sun. Getting our things together, we hurried to the bus and got there just as it arrived.

Bubbles laid on the seat with her head in my lap. I kissed her forehead and stroked her hair. She looked beautiful; her face peaceful as she slept quietly.

Once at Berkeley, we made our way to the Latimer Building and dropped off the compounds with a grad student. She was lovely and told us spots on the campus to visit and wished us an enjoyable day.

We held hands and walked up and down the hills of the Berkeley campus.

We discovered an outdoor cafe, and ordered breakfast. She had an air of elegance as she sat leisurely eating her croissant in the backdrop of the university quad.

We climbed the bell tower and looked with wonder at its sixty-one bells.

We'd been sitting on the grass at the quad eating French fries when the bells began to sound. I took Bubbles' hand and headed towards the tower. The sound of the bells was mesmerizing and we were gripped by their enchantment.

When we reached the tower, we laid in the grass; I held Bubbles close and kissed her; then, still holding her, drifted off to the sound of the bells and being with by her...

CHAPTER FIFTEEN

Thursday, August 2, 1984

My thoughts go back a week ago when Bubbles and I made love. Duran Duran was playing on the record player.

> *Some call it a one-night stand,*
> *but we can call it...*

"Paradise," she sang.

I'd been impatient earlier in the week; we'd come back from Berkeley, and didn't give her the time she needed.

"Am I hurting you?" she said.

"No. Your pussy is hurting me."

"My pussy is part of me."

Finally, I became discouraged, and angry with myself.

"Bubbles, I'm sorry about tonight. I feel like I just wanted you for sex and didn't give you the love you needed."

"That's okay, David..."

"No... It's not. Let's go to sleep now."

I'd promised myself that if I ever made love to her again, I would give her the love she needed.

"You satisfy me," she said. "David, you were right that one time I asked you what kind of lover you are - You are the best!..."

CHAPTER SIXTEEN

Friday, August 3, 1984

Last Monday Bubbles had a dream - She was being chased in a train until the pursuer caught up to her and strangled her with a spiked chain.

"I died in the dream... I think I died. Maybe I woke up just before I was going to die. Yes, I did. It was weird. I saw a girl in the dream who I haven't seen in years - She was my best friend in fourth grade..."

"Was she killed, too?"

"No, she watched me being killed. I called to her and called to her..."

"That's horrible, Bubbles."

"I always have dreams like that. I'm always killed in my dreams. Most of the time I get an ax thrown into my back - That's why my back gets sore."

"I thought you said you liked sleeping, Bubbles?"

"I do. I love it. I could sleep all the time."

"I wouldn't if I had dreams like that."

"I'm lazy."

"No, you're not. You're worked too hard. If you're not working, someone's taking you out until late at night. You don't get time to sleep."

"Oh, I remember how the dream started now... You and I were making love."

"I was in the dream?"

"Yeah. We were making love. Then you said, 'Come on, Bubbles' and I followed you into a tunnel, and you disappeared and I was in this train…"

That Monday Bubbles told me she wanted to be with me. She said she loved me, needed my love, and she wanted me always.

"Bubbles, I'll love you always. I'll love you forever. But right now I can't make you mine. I wish that love could be my first priority, but at this time in my life my studies and research are the most important things to me. And if I were to take you into my life, I could just see myself working like a mad man to do my studies, to do my research, to be with you - And just doing a half-ass job of everything. Bubbles, I love you, but at this time I just can't make the commitment to you that you deserve…"

CHAPTER SEVENTEEN

Saturday, August 4, 1984

I woke up early the Monday morning before Bubbles was to go home. I watched her sleeping. Lying on her back, she was beautiful - Appearing tranquil and lovely as she slept.

Then I noticed the covers on top of us; there'd only been sheets when we went to sleep - She must have gotten up during the night to get them, and carefully put them over me, so not to wake me.

I kissed her; she put her arms around me and held me tight.

"I must look terrible," she said.

"You look beautiful."

"What time is it?"

"About nine."

She stretched her arms.

"Hmm. I'm sleepy."

"Should I put you back to sleep?"

I caressed her breasts.

"Oh, yeah."

She laughed.

"I remember the first time you caressed my breasts - I was scared."

"So was I," I said. "Did you want me to, though?"

"Yes!"

I lowered my head to kiss her.

"How about taking a shower with me?" I asked.

"Well, I don't know."

"Okay."

I stopped the conversation, and caressed her face. She lost all expression, then, suddenly, her face lit up.

"Hey, want to take a shower with me?!"

"Well... I'd love to."

Holding her hand I assured her the water was warm and we got in.

I reached for the soap, lathered her breasts, and caressed her.

She washed my chest and sides. Her touch was firm and reassuring.

She smelled the soap.

"This is Coast," she said. "Wakes you up!"

She began to wildly run the soap up and down my chest. I laughed and cried out, then held her close; the water running over us.

"I like to watch the water run over your face," she said.

I let the water run over my face some more.

"You're gorgeous!" she said. "You're so beautiful. I LOVE YOU."

We got out of the shower and stood in front of the mirror.

She put on her make-up. Pulling me close, she applied mascara to my eye.

"This must really look cute," I said.

"Hold still."

I looked in the mirror.

"Oh, gorgeous."

"Your eyelashes are so long," she said.

"Jealous, huh?"

"Yeah."

"I can't wait to go to the Chem Building looking like this."

"Do you want me to do the other eye?"

"No. I want this one to really stick out - I want to wink at all the professors. Give them the big wink..."

"A double wink."

"What?"

"A double wink. The kind you do when you're a kid and can't wink yet. Like this."

She blinked her eyes back and forth with nodding movements of her head.

I laughed, pulled her close and kissed her.

"You're so cute, Bubbles."

"I'm cute?..."

"Yes," I said with a kiss. "You-are... in-cre-di-bly... cute... I-love-you."

"Well," she said, returning my kisses. "You're beautiful... And-I-love-you-too."

I looked in the mirror at the mascara on my lashes.

"You're so vain, David."

"I am not..."

"Yes you are. Every time you pass by a store with a glass window, you look at yourself. You are vain."

I wanted to tell her it was because of the woman walking with me.

"I'm glad," she said. "You should like the way you look - You're beautiful. It's terrible when people can't stand how they look. I'm vain, too. I'm always looking in the mirror."

I laughed.

"You know what? I think I want to hold you in my arms and love you all day."

"What makes you think I want to be held and love and touched by you?"

"What makes you think I care what you want?"

"Oh, so you're going to force yourself on me?..."

"Until I can't love you anymore - And, baby, that will be a long time."

I held her hand and led her into the room.

I stood naked before her. She slowly took off her shirt, then removed her undies.

She knelt in front of me, looking at me with trusting eyes. I knelt with her.

"David, I love you. I would have never dreamed that I could love you so much. Every day I love you more and more. You're making me fall more and more in love with you. I want you. I want your love always."

"Bubbles, I love you, too. You'll always have my love. I love you so much. I wish I could make love my first priority - But it isn't - I love you, but my studies have to come first. I'm sorry, but I love you too much not to be honest with you."

"David, I don't want to change that. I've always admired that about you. I wish I could sit down and study like you, but I'm too selfish - I like having fun too much..."

"No. You're too giving. You're too giving to people to deny them your time. I'm like that, too. I love helping people - The problem is they're so used to how hard I work that they don't ask me to help very much - It's too bad because I like helping people.

"Bubbles, you tell me. Is there any way it could work between you and me? Is there any way I could still have you and my studies and my research? Tell me, Bubbles, and I'll try. Just tell me, and I'll do everything I can."

She thought for a long time, our eyes never leaving each other.

"David, I don't think there's any way we could make it..."

CHAPTER EIGHTEEN

Friday, August 10, 1984

Monday before our trip to Berkeley, she curled her legs around my waist and lifted me.

"Now I've got you," she said. "You're all mine..."

Earlier in the day we'd come back to her room after dancing in the lab. As I sat on the floor studying, she went about watering the plants.

"David, were you mad at me when I locked you out of the room the other night?" she asked.

"No," I said, my heart filled with joy and admiration for her. "It was an accident. I was just glad you were alright."

"Well, would you be mad if I poured this water down your back?"

"I don't think I'd care," I answered, hardly looking up.

Not a moment later, I experienced the sensation of being wet, and the sound of a splash registered in my head, as, confused, I wondered what happened?

"Are you mad now?"

"No," I said.

Then, with her considerable height and strength, she reached down and lifted me to my feet with one hand, and cocked back the other.

"David, if you don't tell me you're mad at me, I'm going to hit you."

"I'm not mad," I said. "Bubbles, I love you. The little things don't matter. You fill my life with happiness. I don't want to change you. I love you just as you are."

"David, if you would have told me it would make you mad if I poured water on you, I wouldn't have done it. You let me take advantage of you. If you don't tell me about things that bother you, I'm going to keep on doing them, and they'll make you madder and madder."

My gaze directed downward, I stood nodding.

"Until I explode," I uttered, softly.

"You understand what I'm saying?"

"Yes. I promise I'll tell you when something's bothering me..."

I asked if she'd like a body massage? She welcomed the invitation.

I massaged her; kissing her; feeling her lips against mine; hands approvingly running through my hair.

But when the time came, I was limp.

Oh, no, I thought.

I wondered if it could have been because of the way Bubbles had talked before. Did her show of authority make it impossible for me to get it up anymore? I was truly fearful.

"Bubbles, I don't believe this. Not again."

She laughed.

"We'd make a funny couple..."

"Hilarious."

She sat up in bed.

"David. I'll never make love to you again."

"Oh no?..."

"Never."

"We'll see about that."

I laid with her in bed. When I went to kiss her lips, she put her hands in front of me, and forced me to make my way through.

"No, no," she laughed.

Finally, she gave in - Embracing me with her whole body and kissing me passionately. She looked so happy now. So excited.

She was tight, though.

"Bubbles, what happened?"

"Don't you like tight pussy?"

"Not when I can't get into it."

"You're going to have to love me some more."

I continued to joke.

"David, stop making me laugh," she said. "It doesn't matter anyway - I know as soon as you get in, it's going to be so great that I'll loosen up in a second."

She got on top and directed me in. She stretched her legs flat on the bed, then wrapped them around my waist and pulled me up.

"Now I've got you. You're all mine."

"For some reason, I'm not intimidated."

Every time I moved, she let out a sigh.

But the springs were squeaking.

"Bubbles, I think we're going to wake up your neighbors. We better get on the floor. Ready."

I tried to lower us slowly, but we landed with a thud.

"Did I come out?" I asked.

She laughed.

"Yes. You did."

She got on again. Every time I felt close, I pressed against her and kissed her breasts and neck.

"David, you were right that one time I asked you if you were a good lover - You are the best."

"Are you ready to do it again?"

"David, don't you ever get tired?"

"Never."

"Do it from the back."

"How do you do that?"

She turned.

"Just like this."

The sound of our bodies colliding made her laugh. I never thought I could have so much fun...

CHAPTER NINETEEN

Saturday, August 11, 1984

In the moonlight that shone through the dorm window I studied her features. A blue glow emanated from them, the tender light reflecting her beauty. Eyes closed, face without expression, there were no lines or anguish. Her hair - long and black - draped lightly over the pillow, and the light that radiated from her bathed me. Where were her thoughts? Could such tranquility co-exist with reality? Could love exist? Could love be real? Could love give birth to the beauty before me?

Bending low I met her lips, as her arms encircled me and drew me near…

Around noon I heard the lab door open behind me, followed by the sound of gentle footsteps, then arms that descended about my neck and shoulders.

"Whatcha doing?" she asked.

"Not much," I responded, staring at the computer monitor. "It's gonna be a long day."

"Ready for lunch?"

"Let's go…"

The sky was clear and blue, as we rode out to the fields beyond the Physics Building. A blanket spread over the grass, we ate from the picnic basket she'd strapped to the back of her bike. Then, my head in her lap, we exchanged stories of our lives.

"When I was little," she said, "our father took our bikes away… A girl on our block got hit by a drunk driver. When she died, he forbid us from riding our bikes. We were never allowed to ride them again."

She broke off and looked away, but not before I saw a tear well in her eye.

"He cared about you very much," I said.

"He did," she conceded.

She sighed

"My sister, Melissa, got into trouble a lot," she continued. "He would send me with her to concerts and parties, so that I could watch her and report back to him. We'd get there, and she'd take off with some guy, and I'd be left there all alone with all these strange guys looking at me."

Conjuring an image of male figures surrounding her (She looking back with those big, soft, innocent brown eyes), I shuddered.

Then, in that moment, I lost all feeling for myself. It was as though I wasn't physical present – instead, existing only in spirit – and all that mattered was my cherished friend.

I reached to her.

"I feel for you," I said. "I feel for you…"

CHAPTER TWENTY

Sunday, August 12, 1984

Two scenes play in my head.

The first is romantic – Walking with a girl on a stage.

I stop before a row of flowers.

"I do declare these flowers yours."

Hopping over a small fence, I look back with noble smile, carefully pick a flower, and extend it to her.

Then, there's the other scene.

"You're going to do what? Are you out of your mind. Think, man. Get a hold of yourself. For God's sake."

I grip my partner's shirt.

"You've worked so hard. You're so close. Would you throw it all away for some petty face?"

The partner tries to speak. I overpower him.

"Don't tell me that. You're just naive. There's going to be a day when you can pick from anyone. You've got looks. You have personality - And keep on going the way you're going, you'll have success, too. Please, for God's sake, don't blow it - Don't throw it all away…"

CHAPTER TWENTY-ONE

Monday, August 13, 1984

The Sunday of the week that she and I first made love I read Bubbles a poem I'd written when we were still in the dorms – after the day that Professor Hope cursed at me, and I felt so upset, and she saw me from across the cafeteria, and insisted I tell her what was feeling, and then we went out.

I told her I wanted to share it with her. She said she would enjoy hearing it.

I'd put the poem in a box of my things that I'd stored in the lab. I told her I would get it when we went there to dance.

However, entering the lab, I was seized with insecurity, and pretended to have forgotten; instead, putting on the Michael Jackson tape and taking her hand. We'd had a beautiful day together, and both of us were a little light-headed.

But when we finished dancing, Bubbles reminded me about the poem.

"You said there was something you wanted to read me," she said, softly.

I went into my boxes and began looking, as Bubbles quietly waited. The first time I went through them, I couldn't find it. I felt glad - but also saddened because I considered it one of my best works.

I looked a second time – It was there. I sat on my desk; she on a stool in front of me.

"Here it is," I said.

I was still reluctant – apprehensive of her response. Would she think I planned what happened between us?

I read the poem.

Saturday, May 12, 1984
After a day with Bubbles.

Bubbles, you have so much love, so much love for me,
Sometimes, when I look deeply into your eyes I can feel myself
just melt,
Melt in your love, and in the warm feeling you kindle inside of
me.

Bubbles, you kiss me gently on my neck, on my cheek, and then
embrace me with your entire body against mine.
You tell me you love me,
You tell me you're glad for me,
You tell me you enjoyed temple and that we'll have to go again
soon.
I say I love you so much.
I tell you you're wonderful and how much I enjoy spending time
with you.

Bubbles, you give me such a wonderful feeling down deep
inside.
You make me feel like I am beautiful.
You supersede my intensity, and bring out a feeling of such
immense tranquility and love for life.

Bubbles, I feel for you so much.
Life is hard for you, yet you still smile.
Sometimes, I feel helpless, knowing how much I want to help,
and knowing how hard life can be on a person.

Bubbles, you're an angel.
But for some reason,
I don't know why,
You seem to be an angel born for toil and endurance of life's
hardships.
Oh, why, oh, why, so much the victim of love's cruelty?

Bubbles, I do love you.
When you take me in your arms,
I feel myself sinking gently, tenderly into love's grip.
You make me feel alive.

You make me feel loved.

Bubbles, stay with me.
Don't become another casualty in life's game of moving on.
You, your love, means so much to me.
The time I spend with you is time made to stand still,
To bring out in me life's joy,
To make me to see how good life really is,
To make me see how much I love,
How much I love you, Bubbles,
And how much you love me.

I kept my eyes on the paper a long time. I had forgotten how passionate my writing was.

Would she think I planned this? I thought.

Finally, I looked up from the page. In Bubbles' eyes I saw a blend of happiness and sadness.

"I do love you, David. I love you so much..."

CHAPTER TWENTY-TWO

Thursday, August 16, 1984

As the days pass I realize more and more how much I miss Bubbles. Since she's gone away I've felt like a part of me is missing.

The Tuesday afternoon before she left, we were in Julie's spare room, and Bubbles was folding the sheets.

"Bubbles, I want a kiss."

"You do, huh?"

"Yes."

"What makes you think you deserve one?"

Suddenly, even though she was only playing, I was struck with an empty feeling. What did make me feel I deserved a kiss? I had taken her love freely - With no commitment or responsibility. How could I do that to a woman I loved?

I lowered my head.

"Do you think you deserve a kiss?" she asked.

"I don't know," I answered feebly.

She moved forward and seized me in her arms.

"Well, you do!" she said.

She kissed me down my cheeks, and, as I lifted my head, kissed me up and down my neck.

I broke away and stared into her face; there was a look of joy and happiness in her eyes.

"I love you, Bubbles. I love you so much."

"I love you, too, David. You make me so happy."

We held each other.

Dear God, how I love her. How much a source of happiness and love she is.

"You're making me fall more and more in love with you," she said.

She had told me those words on the Sunday we'd spent at Emerald Bay in Lake Tahoe.

Carol had left us to be by herself. Bubbles and I decided to take a swim in the lake.

Bubbles took off her shoes and rolled up her sweat pants.

I put my feet in the water and let out a gasp.

"Bubbles, it's cold."

"You sure you want to go in?"

"At the moment - No."

"Because I'm only going to take off my sweats if we're going all the way in."

I hesitated.

"Take'em off, Bubbles. We're going all the way."

"I only have my undies underneath them."

"Nobody's looking."

"Except you."

"Would you like me to turn around?"

She smiled and pulled my head to kiss my lips.

Holding hands, we went into the water.

Bubbles went ahead of me.

"Take it easy, Bubbles."

She stopped and I slowly advanced to where she was.

"You have a wet cock, don't you?" she said.

"I suppose you could say that," I responded. "And you have a wet pussy to match, don't you?"

She giggled; I was still a little stunned.

"You're so cute. You're so incredibly cute. I just want to kiss you all over."

We went deeper into the lake.

"Do you still want to go in, David?"

"Yes, I'm just having a problem convincing my body of that."

"Just to say we went into Emerald Bay."

"Yep. Just for the hell of it."

"Why don't we just get out and say we did it?"

"Uh, uh. Comes a time when you have to go all the way. Ready, Bubbles, on the count of three, jump."

"Okay."

"One. Two. Three - Jump."

We both dove into the icy water. We rose to the surface smiling and breathing deep.

"This is great," I said and swam and kissed her.

"I know. I love it."

She dove under and swam deeper into the lake. I dog paddled after her.

She rose with a smile and startled expression.

"Oh, it's freezing," she said. "Oh."

She swam past me and onto the shore.

"Bubbles, be careful."

Out of the lake she stood shivering on the shore.

"It's cold out there," she said.

"I believe you."

I got the picnic cloth and wrapped it around her.

"Bubbles, I think you better take off that wet shirt."

"I don't want anybody to see me."

"I'll keep the picnic cloth around you."

I caressed her breasts and shoulders.

"Well, now we can say we did it, David."

I pulled her close.

"I love you, Bubbles."

"I love you so much, David. You're special. David, I don't know what to do. You're making me fall in love with you - You are! You're making me fall more and more in love with you..."

Finally, the time came to leave Lake Tahoe. Carol drove; Bubbles sat in front; I was in the back.

We had some chips and avocado and took turns feeding each other.

I encircled my arms around her, as she lay with her head on my shoulder. I kissed her head tenderly. I felt a feeling of hollowness; but, then, thinking of all the wonderful times we shared, my heart was filled with love.

Then, Bubbles turned around and faced me; her eyes watery.

"I'm crying," she said.

I moved close to her.

"I love you, Bubbles."

"I love you, too, David."

We drove on. It was getting late and the time getting closer to the take-off time for Bubbles' flight.

Carol said her neck hurt, and Bubbles took the wheel and drove. I desperately wanted us to make the plane. I wanted to say good-bye to her today - I didn't know if I could bear seeing her another day. I had my whole speech prepared. I would tell her how happy she had made me and how I would always love her. Now was the time. Hurry, let's make the plane.

I went to sleep in the back. When I awoke, we were stopped.

"Why are we stopping?" I said.

"It's too late. We can't make the plane. It's too far away," Bubbles answered.

Bubbles got out and called the airline. The next plane to Taft didn't leave till Tuesday. She made the necessary flight changes.

"Bubbles, I'm sorry you missed your plane."

"Wouldn't you like me to stay with you?"

I smiled.

"I'd love that, but I want you to be with your family, too."

We decided to make the plane again, but the freeway was crowded and there was no way we could get there on-time.

We got off the freeway and pulled into a gas station. Carol went to a pay phone and called the family in Taft. I sat with Bubbles.

"What do you think you're going to do now?" I asked.

"Love you," she said.

I pulled her close and kissed her.

"I love you. I love you," I said.

Then, suddenly, abruptly, Carol had a change of heart. She wanted Bubbles to leave on a plane - any plane - tonight. She forced her to drive, battering her verbally for not knowing the way to the airport, for not having enough gas, for not driving fast enough, for not listening, and so on.

My blood began to boil. A little while ago it would have been fine for Bubbles to leave. But now she was being forced.

We got lost looking for the Sacramento airport.

"Carol, I'm tired," Bubbles said. "I think I just want to go back to Davis and sleep."

"Don't be silly. You have nowhere to go back there. Keep driving. We're going to see if they have any other flights to Taft at the airport."

I could sense that Bubbles becoming unnerved; I rubbed her shoulder to calm her - To calm me!

Finally, we got to the airport. Bubbles and I got out of the car and went to the ticket counter.

"Bubbles, I'm worried."

"Why, David?"

"I feel like you're being pushed into something you don't want to do."

The person at the counter told us there were no flights to Taft except the one she had booked on Tuesday.

We went back and told Carol, and told her we wanted to go back to Davis. She didn't resist.

Back at Davis, we all went to my Chem lab. I showed Carol around and told her I would get Bubbles a place to stay with a girl I worked with in the lab. Carol was satisfied. She kissed us good-bye and despite my request she stay with us rather than continue driving, left for Concord.

We watched her drive off.

"Bubbles, I want to tell you something. I think you're wonderful. You're so patient - So understanding of people."

"David, I don't think you know me."

"Bubbles, you are."

I kissed her.

"I feel like so many people try to train you - Try to impose their will on you - Try to make you something that you're not - Try to force you to do things that you don't want to do. Bubbles, I love you just as you are. I want you just as you are. I just want to love you for being you. You're so special, so wonderful."

"David, you keep on telling me these things that most people don't think at all. I'm selfish. I am..."

"Yeah, you're so selfish that you take yourself from your studies to see a movie with Stan so he won't be alone; you're so selfish that you see a blood drive and you're automatically moved to give blood. Bubbles, you're the most unselfish person I've ever known. I come back to Davis - I have no place to stay - you can't help but feel for me and want to help me and take me in so I'll have somewhere to sleep. You make me lunches because I don't take the time to eat properly - Bubbles, I can reiterate a thousand examples of your kindness, of your unselfishness, of your generous love. Oh, Bubbles, I'll always remember that night when I came home late from a hard day at the lab, and when I entered the room - even though you had been sleeping - you reached out to me and embraced me with open arms. Bubbles, you'll never know how much that meant to me. I love you, Bubbles, I really do.. You're my favorite person in the world. The most giving, the most loving person I've ever known."

I embraced her.

"Why do you tell me things that no one else does?"

"Bubbles, everyone loves you. Professor Hope is enchanted by you. Julie loves you - she loves how open you are."

Then, out of the corner of my eye, I saw Julie and her boyfriend Bob walking towards us.

"Well, speak of the devil," I said.

"Hi Dave," Julie responded.

"Hi Julie. Hi Bob."

"Oh, Dave, we got something for you."

Bob pulled out a big cowboy hat and placed it on my head.

"Well, thank you," I said.

I looked at Bubbles.

"How does it look?"

She smiled.

"It looks great on you, Dave," Julie said. "My mother tried to give it to my stepfather, but he didn't want it. So she gave it to Bob, but he already has a lot of hats. So we thought we'd give it to you to add a little character to the Chem building."

"I'll definitely wear it," I said. "Oh, Julie, I have a favor to ask. Remember you said you had an extra room... Well, poor Bubbles just missed her plane and she kinda needs a place to stay..."

"Sure, Dave. Will you come, too?"

"If it's alright..."

"Yeah, sure," Julie and Bob said in unison.

Julie did some work in the lab, then we went to Julie's apartment; I told her I deeply appreciated she taking Bubbles and I in.

I kissed Bubbles to sleep. We fell asleep in each other's arms. I could feel myself very much in love with her. I was unsure about the future, but wasn't going to hold anything back...

CHAPTER TWENTY-THREE

Saturday, August 18, 1984

"I love you, David."

She looked at me sincerely. I'd been wanting to tell her that since she'd picked me up at the bus station in Taft, but hadn't found the right moment. Now we were in her room and I was about to read her the poem I'd written for her - But before I could read, she sat down on the bed and declared her love for me.

"I love you, too, Bubbles."

I leaned forward and kissed her.

She got up.

"I really don't want Lizzy to come in here and see us."

She opened the door and went into the living room to get her shoes. I followed her. Her father was sitting in the reclining chair.

"Did you enjoy the water?" he asked.

"Yes, it was great," I said. "That little David is a terrific kid."

"He didn't like the slides too much," Bubbles added. "Davilo was really excited about going, but he was afraid of going underwater at the end of the ride."

"Yes," said Mr. Vasquez. "He was caught under water once and couldn't get out."

"Yeah," Bubbles expanded. "The water wasn't deep, but at the end of the ride he would go under a little, and after three times he wouldn't go in anymore."

"I remember once," I said. "I was afraid to use a knife because I cut myself really badly at the restaurant where I worked. I called to tell my dad I was quitting my joy. He say, 'David, I've never known anyone who gets as many cuts and burns as you. What's a matter with you? - Don't you concentrate? And what are you going to do later? - Have your wife cut your meat for you - even better, have you kids do it for you? When you're in surgery, are you going to have the nurse use the scalpel? You can't run away from your fears. You've got to confront them!' After that, I really concentrated when I used a knife, and haven't cut myself since."

Mr. Vasquez leaned back in his chair.

"Once, a man I knew in Mexico had to kill a pig," he began. "He sent his son to a neighboring farm to ask for the farmer's sharpest knife. The other farmer - well, he gave the son the knife, but told him over and over to tell his father not to cut his nose."

Bubbles and I both had our hands over our noses.

"The boy got back to his father and give him the knife. The father - He sharpened the knife real good. The son - He remembered what the other farmer said. He tell his father that the farmer says not to cut his nose."

"The father picks up the knife and says to his son, 'How am I going to cut my nose? - Like this,'" he said with a corresponding arm movement.

We gasped.

"And he had a big nose, too - Real long. Cut the thing right off...

Bubbles and I left the house and took a walk. The day was hot and dry. The surroundings on the outskirts of Taft looked barren.

"Is that a ranch over there?" I asked.

"That's were animals are kept."

"Oh, I see."

I smiled.

Our hands knocked together, and I took her hand and lifted it to my lips.

Bubbles pointed to a house; she said she and her family had painted and where her first boyfriend lived .

"Bubbles, tell me about this terrible thing you did once."

"What terrible thing?"

"The thing you could never tell me about."

"Oh, that... You really want to know?"

"Yes."

"Okay. I was just talking about it with Paula a couple of days ago. She says she forgives me. It was with Paula's sister, Anne. You see, I was going out a lot with her and her boyfriend, Ronnie. We'd always be going places together. They found this guy for me to go with, Randy. We'd go out all the time. We were having so much fun.

"Well, sometimes, Ronnie would want to do things, and Randy and Anne wouldn't - So I'd go with him because I thought watching things like car racing was fun.

"Ronnie and I began going out more and more. We were having so much fun and we really liked each other.

"Then, one day, he kissed me - And I didn't stop him - And the whole thing got out."

"And that's it?" I asked. "You just kissed him?"

"Yeah. That's all we did."

I held her.

"Bubbles, I just think that's the way you are. I can feel it: In all the times that you've taken my hand, whether it was the day I was upset because of what Professor Hope told me, or the way you took my hand when we strolled the streets of San Francisco. It's just who you are. You're a loving, wonderful human being."

We walked again.

"So, tell me, what happened after that?"

"Ronnie bought me a stuffed animal and wrote a very incriminating love note to go with it. Anne found the note and wanted to know who it was for. She finally got it out of him that it was me. She confronted me - She was so mad. She called me such terrible things. She hated me after that. She still hates me."

I gripped her hand, then lifted it to my lips.

"And that was it? That's what you've been hurting about all these years?"

"Yes. I lost a friend. She was one of my best friends, and now she hates me."

"Bubbles, I'm sorry, but I don't think there's a right and wrong in love. Sometimes people get hurt - There's nothing you can do about it. It's only wrong when you purposely mean to hurt someone. Bubbles, all you did was kiss this guy?"

"That's all we did."

"My God. What you must think of me?"

"That's different."

"What's so different?"

"You told me... Research first and family second."

"'Family'," I repeated. "I don't even mention a wife. Bubbles, I realize now what love for another is. What can I say - Loving you has been the best thing I've ever known. I want that love in my life."

"You've changed a lot of the ways I think about things, too."
You've changed a lot of the ways I think about things, too."

"Like what?"

"Like the way I feel about Tim."

"How is Tim?"

"He's fine. I saw him when I went to Disneyland. I didn't think I was going to like him. I didn't even want to kiss him. I tried to stay away from him at first. But he's a nice guy. He seemed a better friend to Paula than to me. I don't know... David, did you tell anyone about us?"

I hesitated.

"Yes, I did. I told Nick Delaney... I'm sorry, Bubbles. Remember that night I told you I was at Andy's, and I had a dream I was with you, and I woke up kissing Andy. Well, a couple of days later, Nick told me Andy thought I was a faggot. So I told Nick that I had actually been dreaming of you, and I went on to tell him the whole story."

"That's okay. I like Nick."

"Nick told me to tell Andy, but I told him, 'No way...'"

"Andy has a big mouth."

"Bubbles, why are you so worried Tim will find out?"

"Because I remember when Anne stopped being my friend - I felt terrible. I would be crying all the time. My first weeks in Davis I was still crying. People would stop and say, 'What's that girl's problem?' And if Fred were to stop liking me, I think it would be fifteen times worse. I'd be suicidal."

We walked into a field.

"Bubbles, can I tell you something? The first time we made love, there were a lot of things on my mind. I was thinking things like, 'Am I going to be able to study like I used to?', 'Am I going to be chasing women from now on?', 'Is Tim going to find out and get his fraternity brothers to kick my ass?'"

She laughed.

"I don't think he'd do that."

"I'm just saying there were a lot of things I was thinking about. Bubbles, everything seemed to be going so fast..."

"They were going fast - Very fast."

"Bubbles, I've never let myself go like that before."

"Why did you, David?"

"Because there was time. Because I loved you and had always loved you. I can't help it. I love you so much."

We sat on the street corner.

"David, have I hurt you?"

"No, never. Any hurt I've felt has been self-inflicted. You've only brought happiness into my life."

I looked at her.

"Have I hurt you?"

"No. It's the same. I only hurt myself."

She looked at me with gentle eyes.

"Bubbles, I do love you. You're so special. Please promise me something. Promise me you won't settle for second best. You're too good for that, Bubbles. You may hurt people, but, Bubbles, sometimes that's the way life is. People do get hurt. And if you live life trying to please everybody else - Well, you might succeed in pleasing them, but I can promise you that you won't be pleased. I love you so much, Bubbles. You've made me so happy. The thing I want most is for you to be happy."

"David, you told me that I'm unselfish. But you're the most unselfish person I've ever known."

I kissed her.

"Bubbles, you're the most beautiful person I've ever met - inside and out. You deserve the best. You deserve it."

She reached out to me and pulled me close.

"I love you, David."

"I missed you so much over the past weeks. Please, do me a favor - No matter what happens, let me know you love me."

"I will. I'll send you a book. I'll say, 'I love you. I love you. I love you. I love you.'"

"I never thought this would happen. Bubbles, I've always loved you as a friend, but I never thought something like this would come about."

"I've always loved you, David. I never thought anything would happen. I just wanted to be your friend for always. I do love you, David. I wouldn't make love to you if I didn't."

"Bubbles, what did you think would happen at the end of the summer?"

"I tried not to think about it."

"I was the same way. I decided to take one day at a time and let things happen. I did have thoughts, though. I thought you would go back to Fred, and I would just live with the memories. I thought I would love you until it was time to say goodbye."

"I don't want this to be just a summer fling, David…"

CHAPTER TWENTY-FOUR

Monday, August 20, 1984

"David, are you my friend?"

"Yes, I'm your friend."

"Do you just want to be only my friend?..."

She and her sister brought me to the bus station.

"Bubbles, I need some time to think. I love you, though - I'll always love you..."

CHAPTER TWENTY-FIVE

Wednesday, August 29, 1984

A week ago I called Bubbles to tell her I couldn't keep her in suspense any longer. Although I longed to be with her and make her mine, there was too much ahead of me than to make a commitment to a person.

Bubbles replied that she hoped we could still be friends. I told her I would always love her.

I felt bad. But to make a commitment to someone now would only mean heartache and anger at that person if things didn't go as I planned.

And there were her dreams? She wanted to be a veterinarian. I couldn't take her with me and at the same time fulfill that. We'd both wind up broken apart and disassembled in disarray.

Last night I called her again. A man's voice answered.

"Hello."

"Hello Mr. Vasquez. May I speak to Bubbles?"

"Who is this?"

"Dave. Hi Mr. Vasquez, how are you?"

"Oh, Dave. I'll get her."

"Hello."

"Hi Bubbles."

"Who is this?"

"Dave."

"Dave who? I don't know any Dave."

"Oh, no. I guess I must have the wrong number."

"I guess so..."

"Bubbles. I put ninety cents into this phone..."

"Okay. How are you?"

"Fine. When are you coming up here?"

"Saturday I think. My dad's going to take me and help me unpack."

"I need to buy some things for my apartment. How about going with me to San Francisco?"

"How would we get there?"

"Berkeley bus."

"When?"

"Monday."

"I have rush."

"How about Tuesday?"

"I have rush all week long."

"Oh well, I guess you're out of luck..."

"You're out of luck."

"Uh, uh. You are. I'll find somebody else."

"Another girl."

"No. I'll pick up some guy there - It's the place for that kind of stuff."

"Get some bu-fu," she laughed.

"That's uga-buga... And, yeah, that's right."

"I told that joke to Tim - He thought it was a crack-up."

"Well, you must have told it right - I can never get a laugh when I tell it."

"We were saying, 'Yeah, Dave Fischer finally told a funny joke.' We're so mean to you."

"That's alright. I'm used to it. Bubbles, what are you doing on Sunday?"

"I don't know."

"Would you like to have dinner with me?"

"I don't think so."

"Oh, no?!"

"No... I think I'd rather take you to the fair."

"Cal Expo?"

"Yeah."

"How would we get there?"

"We'll get someone's car."

"Great."

"But I have to have money."

"I have money."

"I have to have money, too."

"Alright - If not, we'll go dancing at my lab..."

The operator broke in and asked for another dollar and thirty cents.

"Bubbles, I'm getting off. I love you, but I'm not paying no dollar-thirty..."

"You have to, or else I get charged."

"You do?"

"I think so."

"Okay."

I put in a dollar and twenty cents.

"Operator, that's it - That's all I have."

"I'll accept the rest of the call, operator," Bubbles said.

"Alright, ma'am."

"Good," I said. "Now we can talk as long as we want."

"No way, pal. I don't want to get into trouble, either."

"Okay, then Sunday we'll go to Cal Expo, and San Francisco we'll see."

"Alright, I'll call you on Saturday."

"Good. Or I'll call you. I love you, Bubbles."

"Take care, David..."

CHAPTER TWENTY-SIX

Sunday, September 2, 1984

"Hello, may I speak to Bubbles?"

"This is Bubbles."

"Hi Bubbles."

"Hello David. How are you?"

"Fine. How are you?"

"I'm okay. Hey, where are you? I've been looking and calling for you all over the place."

"I'm in the Chem lab."

"No, you're not. I've been calling there for the past hour."

"I'm at the 7174 number."

"Yes, that one."

"I'm sorry, Bubbles. I must have just missed you. I was out getting some sun..."

"Don't be sorry. I even went out to your place - You live way out there."

"Bubbles, how long have you been back?"

"About an hour. When are you going to come see me?"

"Why don't you come here and see me?"

"Okay. You'll open the door?"

"Yeah. When will you be here?"

"I'm leaving right now."

"I'll be waiting."

"Okay. Bye, bye, David. See you soon."

She has so much love in her heart, I thought. So much love for me.

Tears came to my eyes.

How could I doubt her when she's so wonderful to me?

I went upstairs to Professor Poole's lab to wait for Bubbles. When I saw her, I dashed out, burst through the doors, jumped down the stairs and ran to her open arms.

"Hi David."

I kissed her.

"God, I'm glad to see you. God, I'm glad you're back…"

We rode to my apartment. The place was still unfurnished – just white walls and bare. I went to the kitchen to offer her something. When I returned, she was sitting on the floor, and moved by her quiet grace, poise and humility, I fell to my knees beside her and held her close and kissed her. She pulled off my shirt.

"I want to make love to you, David," she whispered…

CHAPTER TWENTY-SEVEN

Wednesday, September 5, 1984

In the morning I kissed her.

"I want to wake you up every morning with love," I said. "Holding you close to me and showering you with kisses..."

"And sticking your cock up my pussy," she inserted, smiling.

"Oh, Bubbles."

"Well?..."

We showered.

When we finished, I turned off the water, and she took the towel.

"First, your hair," she said, running the towel through it. "Then, you scalp. Then, your eyebrows.

"Then, your nose - The whole towel!

"Your shoulders - Lift your arms, cutie!

"Your arms and underarms. Your chest, your stomach, your belly button. Your cock - Two threads."

I laughed. She was laughing, too. I put my arms around her and pulled her close...

CHAPTER TWENTY-EIGHT

Thursday, September 6, 1984

Bubbles came over to my apartment this afternoon to go swimming. We went into my room and undressed.

Just as she was about to put on her bathing suit, I extended my hand to her. She dropped the suit and slowly walked over.

"David, I can't go swimming."

"Why not?"

"Because I'll smear my mascara," she joked.

I pulled her close.

"Oh, no!" I responded, playful.

"I'm so tired," she said. "We stayed up late last night. I don't think I got to bed till 1 am."

I nodded. Time was running out.

"Bubbles, I didn't expect to make love to you at all when you came back."

"I didn't think we would, either," she responded. "But I wanted to share my emotions with you."

I felt touched.

"I hope we can still go dancing in my lab and do things together," I said.

"You'll still take me to temple on Friday nights? You'll be my pal?"

I looked away.

"Bubbles, I'm someone who loves you."

"I love you, too, David."

She kissed me and held me tight...

CHAPTER TWENTY-NINE

Saturday, September 8, 1984

On Thursday night I was working late at my desk in Professor Poole's lab, when, suddenly, I saw something moving up and down just outside my window.

Bubbles!

I rushed out through the doors and embraced her.

"I was beginning to wonder how long I was going to have to hop up and down before you saw me."

We walked up the entrance stairs, and I pulled out a new set of keys.

"No more having to go through the back for us."

I took Bubbles' hand.

"I have to get the tapes out of the lab."

"Hey, there's my plant. I'm going to leave my keys by it so I remember to bring it back with me to the House."

She put her arms around my shoulders.

"Hey, you know what? I had two glasses of white wine. So tonight you have a very happy Bubbles."

"And, knowing you, they were probably full glasses."

"Nothing goes better with fish than white wine."

"Come on. Let's dance."

I took a detour through the X-ray lab.

"I've had nothing but problems with these crystals - The quality is poor, the scanning is slow, and I have doubts about the axial dimensions."

"What if it's not right?"

"Then I've done the best I could. I'll have someone check it tomorrow. If it's wrong, I'll try again."

"It's a lot of work, isn't it?"

"It can be."

We left the X-ray room and went to my lab.

"Would you like anything to eat?" I asked. "We have some watermelon?"

"Is it sweet, like you?"

"It's sweet."

"I'm still stuffed. Hey, let's dance."

Bubbles and I danced. She pulled me close.

"David, what are you doing to me? I'm so crazy about you."

She hugged me and kissed my neck.

"You're awesome," she continued. "You're so fun. Let's play that song again."

I re-wound the tape.

Bubbles moved closer to me. She kissed my lips and stroked her fingers through my hair.

"I love you, David."

Bubbles hugged me at the song's completion, then looked up when the next song started.

"Hey, we didn't get to dance to that song last time."

"No. We didn't."

"You were too busy raping my lips."

"Let's dance to it."

We danced and twirled and sang to the rhythm and lyrics of the song.

Bubbles went to the water faucet for a drink. I went back to my desk and sat quietly for a moment. Bubbles came over to me and sat down next to me.

"Do you think a lot about the research, David?"

"I suppose."

"It's a lot of work, isn't it?"

"Anything can be a lot of work, especially if you don't know what you're doing. That's something that impresses me about researchers like Professor Poole - he's working with things that have never been discovered. He's a very innovative man."

"What does that mean?"

"It means he's inventive."

"What does he do?"

"Basically, he makes new molecules."

"What's the good of it?"

"To know. To attain knowledge in areas where we know little. Who know? Maybe somewhere down the line his discoveries will have practical applications. But today the driving force for these discoveries is the desire to know.

"My dad asked me the same question - 'What's the good of it?' Just to know. I must say, though, that when and if I do research, I'd like to do something with practical applications - Like cancer research, where you're trying to combat a harmful human ailment that's caused great suffering... Did I ever show you that letter I wrote to Dr. Sanger at the Cancer Research Institute?"

"You told me about it, but I don't think you ever showed me."

"I'll get it."

I went into my backpack, and pulled out a copy of the letter.

"Here it is. I even got it drawn up on official UC Davis paper."

I sat down and scanned the letter.

Dr. Ryan Sanger
Department of Surgery
Children's Hospital Medical Center
Boston, Massachusetts

Dear Dr. Sanger:

I am a student at UC Davis. Several months ago I read an article describing your discovery of an antibody that halts tumor growth. I was captivated by the article, not only because I am dedicated to pursue a career in medical research, but also because the article offers so much hope to those who are afflicted with cancer..

While reading about your discovery, my mind searched the endless realm of possibilities that could become a reality if the hypothesis behind your discovery holds true. Among the possibilities I conjectured was the notion of determining the molecular structure of the antibody, formulating a means of chemical synthesis and mass production, then putting it into the drinking water throughout the world, thereby, insuring the continued circulation of the antibody in the human bloodstream to effect a halt of tumorous growth in all human beings.

I've dedicated my summer to perfecting of my skill in X-ray diffraction. I feel that I am now in a position to successfully determine the molecular structure of your tumor halting antibody.

Dr. Sanger, my desire to work towards discovering an effective cure for cancer is genuine. I am committed to a life of medical research. I am constantly looking for ways to apply the skills I acquire. It is my belief that the capacity for determining the molecular structure of your tumor halting antibody is within our grasp.

Please know that you have my entire admiration. I wish you nothing but success in your continuing pursuits to combat cancer.

Sincerely,

Looking up from the letter I stared into Bubbles' eyes. She was looking at me solemn.

"You have a lot of confidence in yourself, David," she said slowly, seriously. "I admire that. You know what you want to do and you do it. I wish I was more like that."

I lowered my gaze.

"While I was in Florida, I had such a wonderful stay with my grandfather. He literally fell in love with me. You could see it in his eyes. One day he read some of my free verse. He was so impressed. He told me, 'David, what you wrote here some guys spend years writing a dissertation for, and never express what you did.'"

"You do express yourself well, David."

I looked down, then knelt and kissed her.

"I love you, Bubbles."

"I love you, too, David. I'm glad you can confide in me."

Bubbles looked at me and smiled, the love pouring out of her eyes.

"Only good times. This has really been the best summer I've ever had. Only good times."

She held me close, then looked at me.

"I like you, David. I like you a lot."

We sat and talked for a long time. We talked about her dreams - She was constantly being killed. But she told me it wasn't she who was being killed - but, rather, another person who was just like her in all ways yet wasn't her.

"Bubbles, remember how you told me people are constantly misunderstanding you. Like the way your sister Carol calls you 'Miss Perfect'. She says 'Miss Perfect' to you, but you think it isn't true. Could it be that in these dreams the person being killed is 'Miss Perfect' and others people think and say you are. Is that a possibility?"

"It's possible…"

We danced a little longer.

As we were getting ready to leave, I saw her write a note and put it on my desk. I walked over and read it.

I love you.

I care about you.
You're my favorite.
Numero 1.

I wrapped my arms around her.
"Oh, I didn't write 'I like you.' Here."
She wrote it on the top.
We left the lab and rode to her House.
"I'm not ashamed to say I love you in public," she said. "I love you, David..."

CHAPTER THIRTY

Thursday, September 13, 1984

The days pass. Bubbles and I continue to see each other daily, but both of us are getting more involved in our day-to-day lives. My research work has taken an interesting turn when I observed a phenomenon involving controlled thermolysis. Meanwhile, Bubbles is involved in her sorority rush. The only time she has to see me is when she's given two-hour breaks for lunch and dinner.

When I see her, she's usually tired. Rush has taken a lot out of her. Her eyes show how hard things are getting. Yet she still makes time with me even if it's only for a little while.

Last night I invited her over - She didn't have to get back to the sorority till one the next day and we'd finally have some time together.

"It means, though, that I'll have to bring my clothes over," she responded.

"So bring them."

"Maybe if you twist my arm a little."

"I'm twisting it a lot."

"Oh - Oh. Alright. I'll be over in a little bit."

"Great."

"Hey, what are we going to do tomorrow?"

"It's been so long since we just had time to walk and be together. We'll get up in the morning, pick a direction, and walk and sing and dance."

I heard her laugh.

"You're great. I'll see you in a little while..."

When she arrived, I told her I wanted to take a walk to the train station, next to my complex.

"Why do you like train tracks, David?"

"Because they can take you anywhere."

"So can roads."

"Yeah, but there's something romantic about train tracks. They extend for miles without ever giving you a clue where you're going. And trains are friendly - You could always just hop on and take it where it leads you."

I jumped into an abandoned train.

"So where do you want to go, my lady?"

"Do you really want to know?"

"Yes."

"Home."

"And where's home?"

"Wherever my family is."

"Maybe we can take you there."

I extended my hand. She climbed in. She still looked tired.

Returning back to the gully, I leapt over. She was reluctant. I extended my hand to her.

"How do I know what's down there?"

"You don't."

"Then why should I cross?"

"To get to the other side."

"I'm not sure I want to go to the other side."

"You have to - It's the only way back."

"What is there to go back to?..."

Returning to my apartment, she laid on the bed.

"I'm so tired," she said.

"Take off your clothes, Bubbles, and I'll put you to sleep with a body massage."

She took off her clothes and went to the bathroom. I kept on my underwear.

Bubbles has seen me naked before, I thought. There's nothing to hide - Before, now or after tonight.

She brushed her teeth and washed her face.

"Do you have that skin lotion?" she asked.

"Yeah, I'll get it. I'll use it when I massage you."

"Oh, yeah. I have a note for you, David. It's in my back-pack."

She got the note and handed it to me.

David,
Good for:

1 Back massage
1 Lunch
1 Dinner
You're an awesome friend!!
Love, Bubbles

"Thank you, Bubbles."

"We'll check them off as you use them."

She lay in the bed. I poured the skin lotion into my hands, then warmed it by rubbing my hands together. I enjoyed the feeling of her skin. My fingertips tingled as I caressed her.

"David, this really feels good."

As I massaged her hips I heard the sound of fluid moving below.

When I finished her feet, I asked her to turn over.

"Now, I know you must be enjoying this," I said.

"Because I turned over?"

"Yeah - You're not sleepy anymore."

As I massaged her face, her hands caress my thighs.

"Bubbles, do you want to make love?"

"Do you want to?"

"I enjoy making love to you."

"That's not what I asked... Do you want to make love?"

"Yes. Do you want to?"

"I don't know."

My mind was working hard. "Dicks have no brains," I heard my father say.

There was something more important here - There was love. There was trust. And I wanted that.

"Bubbles, I love you. I love you too much to confuse your life."

I kissed her and moved off.

Then I felt her hold me. I caressed her hand with my fingertips, then followed her hand as it led me.

I could feel her tremble inside.

She pulled me over.

"Bubbles, do you want to make love to me?"

"Yes."

"Are you sure?"

"I'm sure."

Her hands caressed me, then directed me inside.

She let out a sigh.

But I became too excited.

I felt bad. I wanted it to last.

Bubbles pulled me close.

"I enjoy the feeling of you inside of me."

She moved under me. Hearing her sighs made me happy.

I looked at her - Head pulled back - Breathing heavy.

I felt close and held her; she trembled.

"I love loving you, David. I love you. I love you so much."

Her movements became wild - Taking me with her.

She trembled and dug her nails in my back.

"David, I love you so much."

The heat from her rose, and her soft thighs encircled my sides.

Feeling close, I pushed down. Her arms wrapped around me - Her insides trembling.

"I love loving you, David. You make me feel so loved..."

We breathed heavy when it was over. I bent low and kissed her body.

"I love you so much, David. You're special to me. I trust you. I'll do anything for you - Well, anything humanly possible..."

Awakening to the morning sun, she was curled around me. I kissed her cheek, and she pulled herself closer to me. I put my arm around her and let her sleep.

When she awoke again, we held each other and talked most of the morning.

We got up and showered. She spun me around and washed my back. She joked that when I wasn't looking she was going to stick something up my butt. I laughed and said I'd probably enjoy it.

THE END...

EPILOGUE

The angst I felt from having left her would drive me and wouldn't let me rest until I'd developed fulfilled my destiny in cancer research, and developed the first selective cancer vaccine, which would effectively launch the science of NeoAntigen Tumor Immunotherapy, now used the world over to help patients with every kind of cancer.

A leg injury (caused by my uncle and leaving me disabled and in chronic pain) would short-circuited my cancer-fighting endeavors.

But, then, the vestiges of the relationship with Bubbles would get me through that, too, and propelled me forward to advance in the science of Energy Medicine – Because every time I connect energetically with a patient, I tap into that unconditional love I knew with her...

ABOUT THE AUTHOR

David Fischer MD PhD is a physician-scientist
whose groundbreaking research at the National Institutes of
Health was the basis for a FDA-approved vaccine for cancer.
Following a traumatic leg injury, he trained in bioenergy and
introduced energy medicine approaches at the National Institute of
Complementary and Integrative Health. Now, a Professor of
Medicine, he cares for the homeless, leads efforts to
combat the opioid crisis and advances integrative
therapies for the treatment of pain.

www.ingramcontent.com/pod-product-compliance
Lightning Source LLC
Chambersburg PA
CBHW032117280326
41933CB00009B/882